BUT YOU LOOK HEALTHY!

JULIET C WILSON

For information on this book please contact the author:
Juliet Wilson
julietwilson@hotmail.com

DISCLAIMER

The author is not a doctor or health practitioner. The information in this book is not intended to replace the advice of the reader's own doctor or medical professional. It is intended for informational and educational purposes only and not for self-treatment or diagnosis. The reader should consult a medical or qualified health professional in matters relating to their health, and with symptoms that may require diagnosis or medical attention. Individual readers are solely responsible for their healthcare decisions. The author does not accept responsibility for any adverse effects individuals may claim to experience, whether directly or indirectly, from the information in this book. The author does not have any financial interest in any of the organisations mentioned in the book. The fact that specific resources have been mentioned, does not mean that the author endorses all of the information they provide or recommendations they make. It is recommended that the reader obtain their own medical advice.

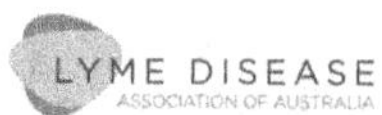

**$1 FROM EVERY BOOK SALE GOES TO
LYME DISEASE ASSOCIATION OF AUSTRALIA**

IN PRAISE OF *BUT YOU LOOK HEALTHY!*

Juliet has skilfully interwoven her own inspiring story throughout a carefully crafted guide for healing complex, long-term disease. Chronically ill patients and their loved ones will find this book to be concise and comprehensive, but by design it is considerate and unlikely to overwhelm those new to the holistic health recovery pathway.

Holding all the information that Juliet painstakingly gathered and utilised to eventually triumph over her debilitating health symptoms, this book has the potential to save patients years of expensive and traumatic searching and suffering, and the frustration of fruitless tests and treatments.

Practitioners of conventional medicine will also benefit from this book, given it includes multiple issues that need to be explored, but are too often overlooked in the diagnosis and treatment of chronic illness. Juliet's personal story, including the psychological suffering that prolonged illness inevitably delivers, is likely to have a lasting effect on those who harbour the tendency to consider ongoing multi-systemic illness to be psychosomatic.

We appreciate that Australian Lyme and associated diseases has been courageously included and examined in this book as a potentially game-changing factor for the chronically ill. For too long, Australian patients and Lyme-aware practitioners and their stories have been ignored, disbelieved and ridiculed. As well as being a valuable guidebook for those lost in the wilderness or at the starting line, But You Look Healthy! represents another significant spanner in the works for the Lyme denial juggernaut.

Lyme Disease Association of Australia

DEDICATION

This book is also dedicated to the passionate and compassionate doctors and health practitioners who made such a difference in my experience along the way.

In particular, I would like to thank Dr. Geoff Kemp, the most outstanding doctor I consulted with in my many years of chronic illness. Dr Kemp has devoted his life to helping Lyme disease sufferers, and to fighting for recognition of Lyme disease in Australia and for treatment for his patients. I believe that Dr. Kemp saved my life, and will always be grateful that I ended up in his office. He deserves recognition for his compassion and selflessness, his encyclopedic knowledge, and for the significant difference he has made to the lives of thousands of chronically ill people throughout his career.

I would also like to acknowledge:

Dr. Anne Small	Judy Meagher, Kineseologist
Dr. Victor Portelli	Dr. Anjana Arunachalam
Dr. Iggy Soosay	Dr. Caroline Baker
Dr Creina Hogg	Dr. Mitchell Chipman
Dr. Mark Hastie	Kate Rogers, Physiotherapist
Carolyn Walker, N.D.	Dr. Martin Harvey
Dr. Angus Pyke	Dr. Kieran Whelan
Anthony Mesiano, R.M.T.	Peter Gibson, N.D.

It is also for my family and loved ones who were loving, supportive, and helped me maintain my sanity along the way, especially David, who checked on me every day from 17,500 km away during the toughest years.

I am not a doctor; I am simply sharing my experiences and the insights I gained along the way. We are all different, and before you start any new treatment protocol, exercise, or supplement speak with your doctor or health practitioner.

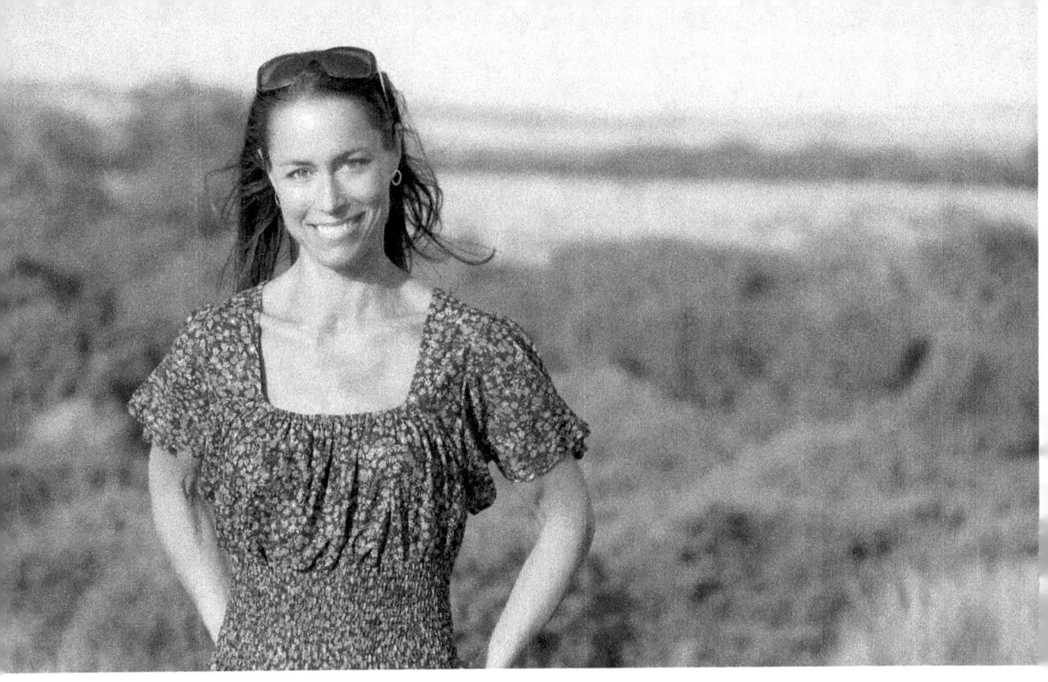

ABOUT JULIET

Juliet survived over a decade of relentless health issues and being told 'But you don't look sick,' by dozens of doctors and specialists, before finally coming across a doctor who recognised what she was dealing with.

Realising that there are so many people like her around the world, not diagnosed properly and struggling for years, Juliet felt it was important to share what she had learned, in the hope of helping others regain their health, and survive the experience along the way.

A senior project manager, photographer, artist and author, Juliet lives with her son in Melbourne, Australia.

TABLE OF CONTENTS

ACKNOWLEDGEMENTS 12

INTRODUCTION BY DR. RICHARD HOROWITZ 13

INTRODUCTION BY DR. GEOFFREY KEMP 19

FOREWORD 27

AUTHOR INTRODUCTION – A COMMON SUITE OF ILLNESSES 31

CHAPTER ONE
GETTING YOUR IMMUNE BALLOON TO FLY AGAIN 37

THE JOURNEY

CHAPTER TWO
ADRENAL DYSFUNCTION
TIRED BUT WIRED 47

What is adrenal dysfunction?
How did I get it?
What are the symptoms of adrenal dysfunction?
The iris flashlight test - an initial indication only
What do I do if I think I have it?
Helpful resources

CHAPTER THREE

HEAVY METAL TOXICITY
WINNING THE LOTTERY 61

What are heavy metals?

What are the symptoms of heavy metal toxicity?

How can I test for heavy metals?

How do I get rid of them?

The pitfalls of detox

Helpful references and resources

CHAPTER FOUR

SMALL INTESTINE BACTERIAL OVERGROWTH
THINGS OVERGROWING IN THE WRONG PLACE 81

What is SIBO?

How do I know if I have SIBO?

Why do I have it, and how can I prevent relapse?

What is die-off?

What are my treatment options?

What is a prokinetic and why is it important?

Helpful references and resources

CHAPTER FIVE

BIOTOXIN ILLNESS
THE CURSE OF LIVING NEAR THE BEACH 99

What is mould illness?

What are the common symptoms?

How do I know if I have mould illness?

How do I recover?

How do I know if there is mould in my home?

How do I safely kill mould myself?

How do I prevent mould?

The connection between mould illness and Lyme disease

Helpful references and resources

CHAPTER SIX

PARASITES
A COMMONLY OVERLOOKED ISSUE 139

How do I know if I have parasites?

How do I treat parasites?

Helpful resource

CHAPTER SEVEN

LYME DISEASE AND CO INFECTIONS
PEELING BACK THE LAST LAYER 149

What is Lyme disease?

Why is Lyme controversial?

What are the symptoms?

How do I know I have it?

Why is Lyme disease hard to treat?

What can I expect when I start treatment?

Helpful references and resources

TRAUMA
AN UNDERLYING FACTOR 165

CANCER
THE BIG ONE 169

TIPS

TIPS FOR SUFFERERS
HOW TO MAINTAIN YOUR SANITY WHEN YOU WANT TO
CURL UP AND GIVE UP 177

TIPS FOR LOVED ONES
TO HELP THOSE CLOSE TO YOU UNDERSTAND WHAT YOU NEED 189

TIPS FOR MEDICAL PROFESSIONALS AND HEALTH PRACTITIONERS
TO HELP YOUR TREATING TEAM UNDERSTAND HOW TO BETTER
SUPPORT YOU 195

CONCLUSION 199

ACKNOWLEDGEMENTS

I WOULD LIKE TO ACKNOWLEDGE THE FOLLOWING PEOPLE, WHO HELPED ME BRING THIS BOOK TO LIFE:

Eliza Jane Wilson, who helped me convey my ideas in the most effective way, Mik Ruff, who transformed my content into a beautiful design, and Dr. Richard Horowitz, Dr. Geoff Kemp, and Dr. Todd Watts, three of the doctors most dedicated to and passionate about helping people with Lyme disease and co-infections recover.

Despite being extremely busy with their mission of helping people, Dr. Horowitz, Dr. Kemp, and Dr. Watts took the time to review my manuscript and give me valuable feedback. May they one day receive the full acknowledgement they deserve for their service to others.

INTRODUCTION BY DR. RICHARD HOROWITZ

JULIET WILSON'S BOOK, 'BUT YOU LOOK HEALTHY!' TAKES US ON A PERSONAL JOURNEY OF MEDICAL DISCOVERY THAT MANY OF YOU READING THIS BOOK WILL INTIMATELY KNOW WELL.

Complex, long-term illness is becoming a common medical complaint which affects hundreds of millions of people worldwide, and unfortunately, the situation is worsening every year. In the United States roughly one out of two people suffers from a long-term medical complaint. Globally, approximately a third of all adults suffer with multiple chronic conditions, adversely affecting their quality of life, and in the case of children, the statistics are *particularly* sobering.

The WHO has determined that 20 - 25% of children and young adults across the globe suffer from a chronic illness, with many of these children dying from that disease. Eighty percent of chronic disease deaths occur in low- and middle-income countries, thereby resulting in not only tremendous suffering for those families involved but contributing to poverty and hindering the economic development of these underdeveloped countries.

To make matters worse, health care costs have continued to rise over the past several decades despite advances in medicine, where 70% of those costs and 80% of the deaths are due to a chronic illness. The diagnosis of a chronic 'unexplained' disease or 'untreatable' illness can therefore be devastating for the individual, family, country, and healthcare system.

The need to find better and more effective solutions for chronic disease is an urgent call to action that Juliet has been forced to address in her journey from illness to wellness. This book is a primer to help guide you or your loved ones to find solutions and avoid the rabbit hole of countless physicians and testing, getting you the help that you need.

For some individuals, the search for answers for unexplained medical illnesses and chronic conditions may not have been fruitful. Stories of bankruptcy and 'giving up hope' are not unusual in this domain. I have heard these stories many times during my 35-year medical career. Although modern medicine has significantly advanced over the last century and discovered answers for a broad range of acute conditions, whether it be advances in robotic surgery, or the discovery of lifesaving antibiotics in the early 20th century, the one area that has been woefully ignored by the health care system is the global rise in chronic disease.

I have personally treated over 13,000 chronically ill individuals during the past 3 decades, who have come to me from around the world after seeing 10, 20, or 30 doctors. They usually have the diagnosis of a chronic fatiguing, Musculo-skeletal illness with neurological and psychological complaints. These patients are desperately looking for answers, and their story typically shares similar threads. Oftentimes, they have gone from doctor to doctor searching for answers, frustrated, spending huge amounts of resources in an attempt to get their life back, which in Juliet's case, she did. She was a mother with an 'invisible illness' living with a young child, and she had to fight for her life and the life of her child. She was forced to become her own medical detective, finding the source(s) of her illness.

Her story is the dilemma of hundreds of millions of people across the globe who look well, but endlessly search for answers for their invisible illness which may be given many names. Chronic Fatigue Syndrome/Myalgic Encephalomyelitis (CFS/ME), Fibromyalgia (FM), long COVID, a non-specific autoimmune illness, early dementia, and Environmental illness (EI)/Multiple Chemical Sensitivity (MCS) are only a few of the common names given to these chronic diseases. These chronic illnesses are a major driver of suffering, health care costs, workforce absenteeism and at its worst, increased mortality. Yet answers are available, and many people do not know they exist. It took Juliet years to discover them, which is why she wrote this book. She is here to divulge her secrets, so you don't have to suffer the same way she did.

What are the secrets that she discovered which are keys on the road to wellness? During Juliet's journey, she discovered that many of the factors that I have seen affect my chronic Lyme population were underlying her illness. After decades of seeing thousands of sick patients, I noticed that there were up to 16 factors which were always underlying their chronic health conditions. I called this model, MSIDS, Multiple Systemic Infectious Disease Syndrome, which I published in two bestselling books and peer-reviewed medical journals. It is equivalent to a patient going to a physician with 16 nails in their foot, asking for relief of the pain, but until the healthcare provider finds and pulls out all of the nails, the patient will not get well.

In Juliet's case, it was some of the usual suspects that I see in my medical office every day. Problems with the gastrointestinal tract, leaky gut and food allergies, environmental toxicity with mould and heavy metals, hormone imbalances and chronic infectious diseases, like Lyme disease. The MSIDS model postulates that inflammation is the underlying cause of all acute and chronic disease, and if we can discover and effectively treat the multiple sources of inflammation and downstream effects, we can help a patient who has previously not been able to get relief.

Whether it be the discovery and effective treatment of multiple infections, environmental toxins, mineral and vitamin deficiencies affecting detoxification pathways, gastrointestinal imbalances, or a chronic sleep disorder, ultimately causing mitochondrial and endocrine dysfunction or low blood pressure, there are answers. The map exists, and it took Juliet many years to discover what I have known for the past few decades. If you work with your healthcare team and use the scientific and medical principles underlying the MSIDS map, some of which are discussed in this book, you can get better.

Hope exists for those with chronic illness, and Juliet's story is one of love, perseverance, and discovery. If you use this book as a general map, utilizing the MSIDS model in partnership with your health care team, you can see positive results and outcomes, helping you get your life back. The philosophy and wisdom attributed to Winston Churchill almost a century ago, now needs more than ever to be applied to chronically ill patients and the healthcare system. "Never, never, never, ever give up… Success is not final, failure is not fatal, and it is the courage to continue that counts".

If you don't give up, and persevere using the hard-earned lessons learned by Juliet, taking along her map and the MSIDS model, you should find the answers that have been eluding you. Have hope. Juliet discovered these answers as have I, and they are now at your disposal to help you get your life and health back on track.

Sending you blessings on your journey to wellness,

Dr. Richard Horowitz

Dr. Richard Horowitz is the author of two best-selling books on Lyme disease *'Why Can't I Get Better? Solving the Mystery of Lyme and Chronic Illness'* and *'How Can I Get Better? An Action Plan for Treating Resistant Lyme and Chronic Illness'* (St. Martin's Press

2013; 2017), as well as a recent cli-fi novel, *Starseed R/evolution*, highlighting innovative solutions for our climate emergency.

Dr Horowitz has dedicated his life to helping and advocating for those with Lyme disease. As well as treating over 13,000 chronic Lyme disease patients from around the world over the last 30 years, he has served as a consultant to government agencies in Australia, China, Belgium, France, the United Kingdom, and the United States, and was given awards from Project Lyme and the Turn the Corner Foundations' Humanitarian of the Year award in recognition of his work.

Dr Horowitz was also co-founder and past president elect of the International Lyme and Associated Diseases Society, and co-authored peer-reviewed international Lyme guidelines. In addition, he has trained over 200 healthcare professionals in diagnosing and caring for treatment-resistant tick-borne illnesses, and was a past president of the International Lyme and Associated Diseases Educational Foundation (ILADEF), a non-profit organisation dedicated to the education of health care professionals.

The Lyme Disease Association of Australia (LDAA) is honoured to have him as Patron, and highly values the strategic counsel he provides.

INTRODUCTION BY DR. GEOFFREY KEMP

DR. RICHARD HOROWITZ, ONE OF THE MOST SOUGHT-AFTER LYME DISEASE DOCTORS IN THE WORLD, IS TO BE THANKED AND CONGRATULATED FOR HIS DEDICATION AND GENEROSITY TOWARDS THE PEOPLE OF AUSTRALIA, AND FOR TRAVELLING TO AUSTRALIA TO SHARE HIS INVALUABLE KNOWLEDGE AND EXPERIENCE AT THE 2016 SENATE INQUIRY INTO A LYME-LIKE ILLNESS IN AUSTRALIA.

Dr. Richard Horowitz, one of the most sought-after Lyme disease doctors in the world, is to be thanked and congratulated for his dedication and generosity towards the people of Australia, and for travelling to Australia to share his invaluable knowledge and experience at the 2016 Senate Inquiry into a Lyme-like illness in Australia.

Unfortunately for Dr Horowitz, he had unwittingly become enmeshed in the non-recognition of Lyme-like disease as a clinical reality in Australia by many specialists in clinical microbiology and pathology. In fact, the report of the inquiry proceedings records the rejection of Dr. Horowitz's advice and the discourtesy to which he was subjected by specialists, who were angry that their knowledge and insights were being challenged.

That he was moved to contribute to Juliet's book is a tribute once more to his abundant good nature and kindness toward humanity, his commitment to have Lyme recognised for the debilitating disease that it is, and to Juliet's great gifts as a communicator.

I commend Juliet's beautiful and comprehensive book describing her experiences, and her practical advice on how to deal with them. It breaks my heart when I meet patients like her, who struggled for over a decade with the debilitating symptoms from a common and treatable disease before I was able to give her an accurate diagnosis. Sadly, Juliet's experience is not unique, and I feel her book can help many people.

My interest in chronic illness began 1978, when our 2-year-old son Andrew developed a juvenile psychosis and a severe sleep disorder after a severe head injury. After five years of managing his psychiatric condition, where he was unable to look us in the eye and learn normally, I became aware of Canadian psychiatrist Dr. Abram Hoffer's work, where he resolved many cases of psychosis with high dose nicotinic acid, and vitamin C. After only four days of putting his treatment recommendations into effect, we regained eye contact with Andrew, and it has never been lost. He subsequently attended a normal primary school, completed the Duke of Edinburgh award at Year 12, has had full-time employment throughout his adult life, married and had a little girl.

Through this experience, I developed an interest in unsolved mysteries associated with chronic disease, and an understanding that you don't have to be a medical specialist to make break-through discoveries. As a GP, I was able to resolve my son's psychosis, after the doctors at the highly regarded Royal Children's Hospital of Melbourne, who had overseen his illness for five years, were unable to.

In the late 1980's, I learned of the role Mycoplasma plays as a cause of chronic rheumatoid arthritis, with remarkable cures described by Professor Thomas MacPherson Brown. In the late 1990's, I learned of Rickettsiosis and Q fever, described by Dr. Cecile Jadin, as causes of chronic fatigue and other long lasting, chronic complications such as rheumatoid arthritis, severe depression, and endothelial lesions. Using this knowledge, I had remarkable favourable responses with long-term antibiotics in my patients who suffered from these illnesses.

My first known encounter with Lyme disease occurred when an academic botanist from Lyme, Connecticut, USA came to Melbourne University around 2010, and gradually developed troublesome and distressing neuralgia.

He owned a forested property near Lyme, where everyone knew about Lyme disease. While living there, he would have occasional attacks of sinus trouble for which he was prescribed antibiotics. After living in Melbourne for a couple of years without further sinus attacks, when he developed neuralgia he concluded that it was caused by chronic Lyme disease, and that he had not developed it earlier because of the antibiotics he was prescribed for the sinus attacks.

He consulted five or six clinical microbiologists, and all of them attempted to deal with the problem in the same way. They each arranged an ELISA test for Lyme disease, which on each occasion was negative. Despite the convincing hypothesis that he put forward to them, that he had chronic Lyme, they did not feel they could treat his condition on the balance of probabilities.

Anticipating a sceptical response from me as well, he came armed with a book called 'Bulls-eye –Unravelling the Mystery of Lyme Disease', by Jonathan A. Edlow, a Harvard University Hospital Associate Medical Professor. It set out the history of Lyme disease in the USA, as well as the persecution of doctors, such as Dr. Burrascano, by the New York State Medical Board. He also provided a medical paper on Lyme disease and its tendency to cause neurological symptoms, and a proposed medical protocol involving the use of long-term tetracycline hydrochloride developed by Dr. Sam Donta, a respected clinical microbiologist located in Massachusetts.

I read the material he provided to me. It made sense, and I provided him with a prescription for the medications along the lines of the Dr. Donta protocol. Three months later, after having experienced the expected flare in his symptoms due to 'die-off' of the bacteria, he returned to thank me for healing his illness. His neuralgia had resolved.

In June 2015, I was consulted by a gentleman who had become increasingly sick and disabled over a period of fourteen months.

His symptoms, after being bitten by a spider in his woodshed, began with a burning neuralgia in his left little finger and arm, head, and neck pain of excruciating severity, bleeding from the bowel, episodes of complex partial seizures and of full epileptic fits, and cardiovascular crises where his pulse rate fell to less than 40 beats a minute. He feared that he might die, and had made provisions for such an outcome.

A neurologist at the Alfred Hospital and a Professor of Neurology at the Austin Hospital were both unsure of what was causing his distress, because the complex multi-systemic nature of his illness lay outside their clinical experience.

Because of my considerable experience in investigating and treating so many other patients with complex, widely varying symptoms over the preceding twenty years, I arranged for him to be tested for tick-associated poly-organ syndrome in Germany and the USA, as well as Australia. The tests in Australia were negative. But the tests for Lyme and associated co-infections were positive in both Germany and the USA. I administered intravenous antibiotics to my patient, which brought him back from the verge of succumbing to a life-threatening illness.

By then, I had treated over 400 cases of Lyme-like disease.

However, things took a distressing turn three months later, when I was subjected to a hearing by the Medical Board of Australia, and prohibited from treating Lyme disease patients. This was despite helping so many extremely sick patients recover their health, and many of them providing testimonials stating their belief that my treatment saved them from dying of their illnesses.

I was not the only general practitioner to suffer this sort of vexatious abuse; six other colleagues were also reported and prevented from continuing to treat Lyme disease-affected patients. Instead of a genuine campaign to protect the public, this appeared to be an attempt to protect specialists' turf. The outcome of the restrictions placed on those of us treating Lyme disease did not protect patients, it deprived them of the only doctors prepared to listen to, investigate, and treat their distressing and occasionally life-threatening illnesses.

The 2016 Senate inquiry was the result of one my patients' bravery and determination after my diagnosis saved his life. He wanted to ensure that the pandemic of Lyme-like disease in Australia was no longer ignored, and that the doctors recognising and treating it were not attacked. He shared his concerns with the idealistic and compassionate Federal Senator John Madigan, who listened carefully and set up two Senate inquiries - one into the possible presence of a Lyme-like illness in Australia, and the other (with then Senator Nick Xenophon) into The Australian Health Practitioner Regulation Agency (AHPRA) and the bullying of doctors through the medical complaints process.

Unfortunately, as of March 2022, the recommendations made in the Final Report of the 2016 Senate Inquiry into Lyme-like Illness in Australia have never been actioned properly. This means that for patients like Juliet, being properly diagnosed and getting access to appropriate care and support is still challenging.

I commend patients like Juliet who keep searching until they find answers, and when the medical system lets them down, seek support elsewhere in their fight to regain their health.

"Those who are healed become the instruments of healing", A Course in Miracles, **Dr Helen Schucman.**

 May this be proven true for those of you who need healing from distressing, chronic illness, and find it, through Juliet's sage advice.

Dr. Geoffrey Kemp

'CHRONIC ILLNESS.
NO ONE GETS IT
UNTIL THEY GET IT.'

UNKNOWN

FOREWORD

IN MY LATE 20S, A PSYCHIC TOLD ME I WOULD STOP WORK WHEN I WAS 39. I HOPED SHE MEANT I WAS GOING TO RETIRE WHEN I WAS REALLY YOUNG.

I let images of walking on endless beaches and travelling the world drift through my thoughts. But I laughed it off, as it seemed unlikely that I would retire so early. I was no longer running my own business that barely fed me, I hadn't invented anything fabulous, and I was aiming for a career in the museum world, where you were lucky to get a volunteer position after post-graduate study. So, I quickly dismissed her prediction, and went on with my life.

Years later, as my world collapsed, her words came back to me. At 39, I was so ill that I had no choice but to stop work for two years as I slowly recovered. I had never dreamed that this was what she had foreshadowed.

Over the next decade, as my health issues became more complex, in spite of everything I maintained the belief that I would be one of the health success stories that I occasionally read about, where people made a full recovery after years of bizarre and varied symptoms. I promised myself that when I eventually recovered, I would write a book, to help others who might be suffering from a similar suite of illnesses.

Well, I finally did. This book covers my journey, and the things I learned along the way.

It was after hearing a podcast about how the trauma of dealing with a chronic long-term illness is compounded further by doctors, and by family and friends who are unsympathetic or disbelieving, that my ideas formed. For me, the podcast resonated deeply. It got me thinking about the many and multi-layered traumas that occur because of being so sick for so long.

On top of dealing with dismissive doctors who trivialised my level of illness, losing my job in my first round of illness, and losing friends and relationships and my healthy, active life all left me feeling lost, isolated, and defective. In addition, I was struggling with the financial stress of the appointments and supplements that kept me functioning.

For many years, I suffered in silence at work because I feared losing my job again, and I worked extra hard to appear to be competent. For a couple of those years, I hung on by a thread. I locked myself in a small meeting room at lunchtime so I could cry and nap, and make it through the afternoon.

Sadly, my experiences are not unique. I wrote this book in the hope that you can recognise your own or a loved one's journey in mine, and that reading my story gives you the confidence that you will find the answers that you need to get well too. I wanted to share the kind of simple, practical, comprehensive information that I wish I'd had access to along the way, written from the perspective of what a patient would want to know. I hope the resources help you to feel informed and empowered, and that using them improves your experience.

I also wanted to share the insights I gained, after realising that we can't expect the people around us to understand what we are experiencing, and that they need guidance as to what support we need. Their journey is difficult and stressful too.

Please note that although I do refer to some of the treatments that I have used, and that are available, I have deliberately not made specific recommendations, as what works for each person will vary depending on their constellation of symptoms and illnesses/ infections, and I am not a medical professional.

'YOU NEVER KNOW
HOW STRONG YOU ARE
UNTIL BEING STRONG
IS THE ONLY CHOICE
YOU HAVE.'

UNKNOWN

INTRODUCTION
A COMMON SUITE OF COMPLEX ILLNESSES

IF YOU HAVE AN ILLNESS SUCH AS ADRENAL DYSFUNCTION, HEAVY METAL TOXICITY, FIBROMYALGIA, SIBO, BIOTOXIN ILLNESS, OR LYME DISEASE, THERE IS A GOOD CHANCE YOU MAY ACTUALLY HAVE A WHOLE SUITE OF THEM.

It took me 12 years to become aware that that when your immune system becomes compromised due to an untreated, underlying illness such as Lyme disease, it is very easy to contract other illnesses and infections. Because so many of them have similar symptoms, it can be easy for some of them to go undiagnosed for a very long time. Each of these is a burden on your body, and cumulatively, they can wreak havoc. I realise now that you will only recover when you remove all of the toxins, pathogens, and infections in a holistic way. This can save you many years of suffering, and will lead to lasting health.

Dr. Richard Horowitz, MD, has given a name to this suite of illnesses – Multiple Systemic Infectious Diseases Syndrome (MSIDS). In his book, *How Can I Get Better? An Action Plan for Treating Resistant Lyme and Chronic Disease*, Dr. Horowitz talks about how millions of people are diagnosed with chronic fatigue or fibromyalgia, and how these diagnoses are often made on clinical criteria, due to a lack of reliable diagnostic tests. Over time, he had noticed that the symptoms his chronic fatigue, fibromyalgia, and autoimmune patients were experiencing were the same as patients diagnosed with Lyme disease.

He put two and two together, and found that when he treated patients holistically for MSIDS, who had not improved with classic treatments for chronic fatigue, fibromyalgia, and autoimmune diseases, they improved. He uses the perfect analogy in his book of how if someone went to the doctor with sixteen nails in their foot, and the doctor only removed one or two of them, the pain wouldn't stop. When I read this, the penny dropped for me.

It had been scary for me to be so unwell for such a long period of time with a range of odd, relentless, and increasingly more debilitating symptoms that no one could explain. As most doctors are taught to only look for one cause of an illness, when someone like me presented with dozens of bizarre symptoms that didn't easily fit the profile of any one disease, it was easy for them to assume some of them must be in my head.

Thankfully, I found doctors and other health practitioners who knew about, tested for, and diagnosed illnesses that weren't name-brand, but which made sense of my symptoms. Their 'integrative' approach was to combine conventional medicine with evidence-based alternative approaches, not to provide band-aid solutions, but to find the root cause of my suffering. While this was very helpful, after many years of various treatments I was still very unwell, and my instincts told me something remained undiagnosed.

For me, getting to that final comprehensive diagnosis took more than a decade. After recovering from my first health 'crash', and a three-year respite, I crashed again. Then again two years later. Each time I had a 'flare', and added an additional diagnosis to the list, it felt like a victory. Each time, I thought I'd found the root cause behind the previously diagnosed illnesses.

It was only after experiencing this cycle over and over, not feeling better year after year, and stacking up diagnoses like a tower of building blocks, that I finally found a doctor who I believe saved my life. He recognised my constellation of symptoms, and diagnosed me with Lyme and co-infections, and MSIDS. At last, I wasn't the 'extreme' patient. He helped me see that what I was experiencing was quite common, though rarely treated properly, and that there was hope ahead.

From him, I learned that many people with autoimmune issues, heavy metal toxicity, gut dysbiosis, biotoxin illness, and Lyme disease rarely have only one of these illnesses. Because of their opportunistic nature when your immune system is low, and the synergistic way they work together, when you have one of these illnesses, you will likely have a few or all of them. It turned out that I had all of these, plus a lengthy list of Lyme co-infections including Babesia, Bartonella, rickettsia (Queensland tick typhus, Rocky Mountain spotted fever, and Murine typhus), H. pylori, Ehrlichia, and blastocystis, among others.

When I look back, there were signs of a compromised immune system early on. It took me nearly a year to recover after having glandular fever (mononucleosis) as a teenager. I have always needed more sleep than anyone else, have always caught every virus and bacterial infection that came anywhere near me, including shigellosis, H1N1, Klebsiella, Campylobacter, and Streptococcus, and had them worse than anyone else. I have always been told by my doctors and practitioners that I had the 'worst reactions they'd ever seen' to treatments.

It seems that contracting Lyme disease at a young age had impaired my immune system, and over time, left me unequipped to fight off anything else.

THIS BOOK OUTLINES MY PERSONAL JOURNEY THROUGH COMPLEX, LONG-TERM ILLNESS TO WELLNESS, AND GIVES INSIGHTS ON HOW TO SURVIVE THE EXPERIENCE. IT IS WRITTEN FOR FELLOW SUFFERERS, THEIR LOVED ONES, AND MEDICAL AND HEALTH PROFESSIONALS.

Much more than just a personal journey, each of 'The Journey' sections provide helpful, practical, easily digestible information for each of the main illnesses I was diagnosed with, as well as common pitfalls to avoid during treatment.

The 'Tips' sections bring together the approach and mindset that helped me get through the many years I was unwell, including chapters on what sufferers need from loved ones and the people that diagnose and treat them, to improve their experience along the way.

At the end, there is a list of the most helpful resources I found.

I hope that this book helps you gain the knowledge of how you can also get well, and helps you believe that you can.

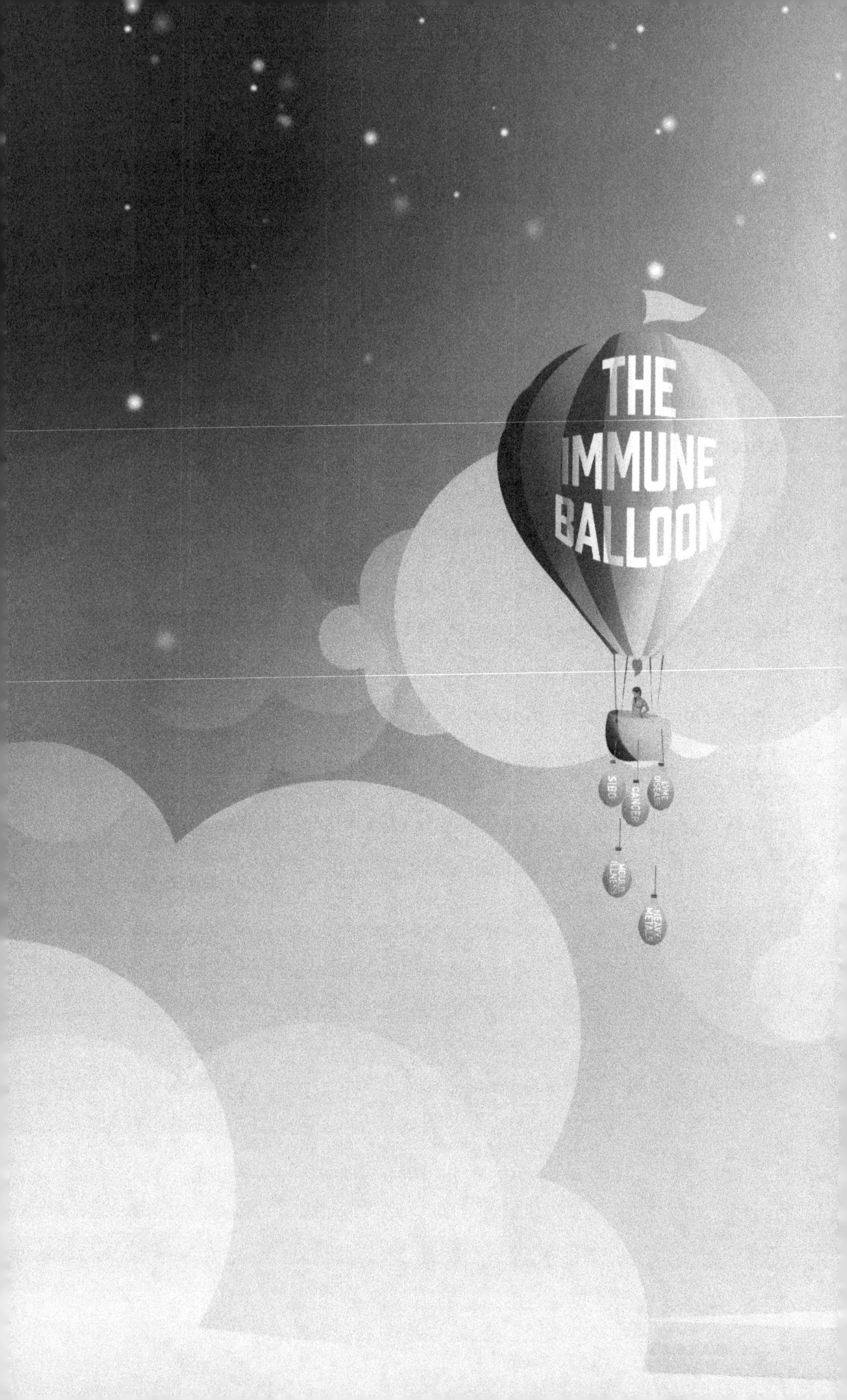

THE IMMUNE BALLOON
SIBO
CANCER
LYME DISEASE
MOLD ILLNESS
HEAVY METALS

CHAPTER ONE

GETTING YOUR 'IMMUNE BALLOON' TO FLY AGAIN

ON TOP OF THE STRESS, PRESSURE, AND NON-STOP PACE OF OUR MODERN LIVES, WE ARE UP AGAINST UNPRECEDENTED LEVELS OF POLLUTANTS, TOXINS, CHEMICALS, AND PATHOGENS. THE CUMULATIVE EFFECT OF THESE TOXINS IS DEVASTATING. COMPLEX, LONG-TERM ILLNESS IS COMMON, AND MILLIONS OF PEOPLE HAVE BEEN UNWELL FOR MANY YEARS AND UNABLE TO FIND ANSWERS.

Last year, I saw a drawing on the cover of an article written by C.L. Jadin in 1999, that stopped me in my tracks. It depicted a gentleman dropping a weight out of the basket of a hot air balloon. Seven other weights remained attached to the balloon and were labelled with other things that can affect our health, like cancer, stress, and pollution, with the label 'Immune balloon' beneath.

I thought it was a brilliant visual metaphor for our immune system, and how each illness and pathogen you collect acts like one of the weights that holds a hot air balloon to the ground. Collectively, they can stop it from flying at all.

To recover and get your 'immune balloon' to rise in the air again, you need to remove those weights. The more you remove, the more easily and better you will fly. Those weights may be SIBO, parasites, fibromyalgia, heavy metal toxicity, mould illness, Lyme and coinfections, undiagnosed cancer, or many other toxins or pathogens. As you remove each one, the burden becomes lighter, until you unload enough of them that your immune system can work effectively, and your balloon can rise into the air and fly.

It is important to understand that detox is a marathon, not a sprint, and going too quickly could leave you feeling worse than before. Although you may want to get rid of the toxins as fast as possible, doing so can backfire. Speed is not important, forward is forward. Go at the pace your own body can handle.

After my diagnosis, as well as when I read Dr. Horowitz's book, *How Can I Get Better? An Action Plan for Treating Resistant Lyme and Chronic Disease*, another major turning point in my journey back to wellness was discovering a company called Microbe Formulas, founded by two doctors in 2017, Dr. Todd Watts and Dr. Jay Davidson. (Microbe Formulas also has a practitioner brand, CellCore Biosciences.) Dr. Todd's success in overcoming his own complex, long-term health issues, and Dr. Jay's success in helping his wife overcome Lyme disease, autoimmune and other health issues, drove them to develop and perfect the supplements and protocols which now help many others.

What sets the Microbe Formulas/CellCore Biosciences treatment protocols apart is that they combine effective supplements with a specific approach. Through research, Dr. Todd and Dr. Jay had gained the knowledge that recovery is more successful, and people will experience fewer side effects, if they follow a particular order to their treatment protocol. Knowing this, they developed the treatment protocols, and there are testimonials from many people around the world who have recovered from chronic illness through using them.

The Microbe Formulas website's 'Learn' section provides numerous resources that explain the order in which to do the treatment protocol, why it is important, and how it works. These resources are searchable by topic, and the Microbe Formulas support team is knowledgeable, and helpful, and is always happy for you to phone and ask questions.

After discovering Microbe Formulas, I devoured every video, article, and recorded webinar on their website. I joined the private Facebook group for people using the same protocol, and suddenly had a community of people like me around the world to connect with, answer my questions, and offer advice. Finally, with a comprehensive diagnosis, an effective protocol to deal with it, and the support of the Microbe Formulas resources, I could see a light at the end of the tunnel. After only four months on the Microbe Formulas/CellCore Biosciences comprehensive treatment protocol, I started to feel significantly better, and after a year I knew I was on the right track to regaining my health.

It is important to note that I do not have a financial gain from this company (or any others mentioned), but also that these protocols may not necessarily eliminate all of the bacteria, because of how bacteria like Lyme persist in biofilms and persister forms, so it is important to work with an experienced medical professional to address your constellation of issues.

The blessing that has come from this journey is the opportunity to share what I learned, in the hope that it can help others avoid years of ill health and trauma.

Hang in there, you can fly again. With the right guidance from a skilled and compassionate team and an effective treatment protocol, you too can recover from complex, long-term illness.

HOW YOU CAN RECOVER

The key to healing from adrenal dysfunction, heavy metal toxicity, digestive issues, biotoxin illness, Lyme disease, and any of the other illnesses that make up MSIDS, is the approach. If you follow these steps, you too can recover.

STEP ONE
SUPPORT YOUR DRAINAGE PATHWAYS

First you need to prepare your body so that it can manage the detox. To do this, you need to open your drainage pathways so that toxins and waste can leave your body. As mentioned, when toxins are not eliminated, they accumulate and can contribute to chronic illness. As well as making your detox more effective, supporting your body's ability to move unwanted things out of your body will also reduce the side-effects (also known as herxing) that you will experience along the way.

SUPPORT YOUR IMMUNE SYSTEM AND MITOCHONDRIAL FUNCTION, SO YOUR BODY CAN DEAL WITH THE MOBILISED TOXINS AND REBUILD YOUR DAMAGED TISSUES AND IMMUNE SYSTEM

Your body will need energy for good drainage and support for your immune system during the detox process. So, it can be important to add in mitochondrial support to give your body the energy required to enable detoxification and for your immune system to fight the infections you have.

REMOVE THE INFECTION, PATHOGEN, AND TOXIN OVERLOAD

Now you are ready to remove the weights that are compromising your immune system. This includes using herbal or pharmaceutical treatment to clear parasites, infections and other environmentally acquired illnesses such as heavy metal and mould toxicity.

USE BINDERS FOR SAFE EXCRETION

The last and essential step is binding up the unwanted elements and by-products released through your detox, so they can be excreted safely. This is done most effectively through using fulvic acid and carbon-based binders, as detailed in Chapter 3.

MAINTAINING YOUR LONG-TERM HEALTH

How do you keep your immune balloon flying high in the future? After removing infections, toxins, and pathogens, giving your body the best chance to stay healthy is a vital aspect of maintaining your new-found health.

You can do this by:

- reducing toxin exposure in your home, food, air, and water
- supporting your immune system
- doing periodic maintenance treatment
- making mental health a priority
- getting enough, restful sleep
- exercising regularly
- eating nutritious food
- minimising stress
- having meaning and purpose in your life
- keeping a hopeful mindset in times of adversity
- remembering that resting is not laziness, it is nourishment.

THE JOURNEY

'COURAGE ISN'T
HAVING THE STRENGTH
TO GO ON; IT IS GOING
ON WHEN YOU DON'T
HAVE THE STRENGTH.'

THEODORE ROOSEVELT

CHAPTER TWO

ADRENAL FATIGUE
TIRED BUT WIRED

I STILL REMEMBER THE FIRST NIGHT I LAY AWAKE ALL NIGHT. IT WAS THE NIGHT BEFORE SELLING OUR FAMILY HOME AFTER THE BREAKDOWN OF MY MARRIAGE. MY ABILITY TO AFFORD THE APARTMENT I HAD FOUND FOR MY SON AND ME DEPENDED ON THE AUCTION RESULT.

The symptoms came on almost overnight. Five kg of weight melted off my already-small frame, my hair fell out in handfuls, crushing exhaustion and insomnia took hold, heart palpitations woke me at 4:00 am every day, and my hormone levels plummeted. Every meal caused digestive distress. I was tired but wired.

Fortunately for me, after a GP told me I was just depressed and tried to put me on Prozac, I came across a wonderful integrative doctor, who recognised what she saw. With almost non-existent estrogen and DHEA, and cortisol that was super-high at 4:00 am then super-low all day, it seemed like textbook, stress-induced adrenal dysfunction (aka adrenal fatigue). The good news she delivered was that because I still had some cortisol production, I would eventually recover.

Then she explained that it might take me two years of being off work to recover fully. The reality of that slapped me in the face. My symptoms made it challenging enough to get through each day. The two years ahead felt daunting.

Adrenal dysfunction was still not widely understood or recognised by conventional medicine in 2008. My doctor had to call it nervous exhaustion on my temporary disability insurance application, for it to be accepted. The saliva testing she used to check my cortisol levels and the bioidentical hormones she prescribed, though widely used now, were controversial then. The other doctors I saw at the time tried to tell me that adrenal dysfunction did not exist and discredited what they believed were dodgy testing methods and snake oil treatments.

I can't even remember the first year, and don't I know how I coped. By some means, I found the strength to be a good parent to my gorgeous 5-year-old. He was the single reason I found the fortitude to put one foot in front of the other.

I was like an overstimulated baby, the more noise or music, bright lights, or crowds that I had to be around during the day, the more overwhelmed and tired I felt, and the harder it was to sleep. Every morning, I woke to crushing exhaustion from not enough broken sleep. Intense brain fog made it difficult to remember simple things and trying to find the energy to do what I needed to as a parent was overwhelming. Stress affected me more, I caught viruses easier, and I felt completely depleted and rundown. My blood pressure was low, and my vision became blurry when I was tired. I had gone from a healthy, active, competent parent and professional to someone I no longer recognised.

It took three years for me to slowly crawl back to feeling like I had normal energy levels, to sleep well enough to regularly pull all-dayers, and for my brain to regain its function. After the first year, it was clear that I was still far from well or being able to work. When my employers at Melbourne Museum found out that I would not be able to return for another 12 months, they said they could no longer hold my job.

The blow was crushing, and broke my heart. Passionate about my work, I had given it my heart and soul for ten years. The last thing I had worked on was the first large-scale exhibition of Australian design. I had helped conceive of, found funding for, and managed the development of this exhibition, which had toured Australia and then had shown in Milan to great acclaim. The Victorian government, the Australian design community, Museum Victoria, and the NSW organisation we partnered with were pleased. The exhibition gave Australian design a prominence that had not been recognised before, created export opportunities for Australian designers, and gave the Museum the younger audiences it wanted to attract.

I thought I would work at Melbourne Museum for the rest of my life. My colleagues were like family, and my son had practically grown up there and called it 'Mummy's Museum'. Feeling like the rug had been ripped out from beneath me again, I was devastated. The only thing that had been getting me through being so ill was knowing I would get back to the work and life I loved once I recovered.

I knew my dismissal was unfair and was encouraged by the Fair Work Ombudsman to take the Museum to a tribunal hearing. Doing so didn't feel right though, and I decided not to go down that path; I didn't need more stress.

With my whole family living overseas in Canada, my income protection only providing 30% of my usual wage, and my medical costs rising above $1000 per month, the road ahead was daunting.

On top of the trauma of losing my job, some of my friends were sceptical of the severity of my symptoms, took it personally that I wasn't being social, and stopped making contact. Although I appeared happy and smiling when I picked up my son up at school each day, they

had no idea the effort it took me just to walk ten minutes to school, or what the other 95% of my day and night was like.

Financially crippled, I couldn't afford my mortgage and had to rent out the new home that had symbolised my new life. I refinanced my mortgage to pay my medical costs for the first of many times. I rented a little house an hour out of the city and began the long road back to good health. I was isolated and alone, but I found beauty in each day, and pointed myself towards the dim light at the end of the very long tunnel ahead.

After two years, I was able to work, and after three, I finally felt good again. I thought that because I had recovered from what seemed to be situational stress, I would never be that sick again. Little did I know that this was just the beginning of a health rollercoaster, and that getting off that rollercoaster would eventually take more than a decade.

I eventually learned that adrenal dysfunction and fatigue issues are a sign of mitochondrial dysfunction. The regulation of hormones happens at the mitochondrial level. Any time there is a threat or perceived threats such as infections, toxins, physical and psychological trauma and other environmental stressors, your mitochondria enter 'cell danger response'. When this natural and intelligent survival response is activated, instead of staying inside your cells and producing energy, your ATP (adenosine triphosphate) leaves your cells, acts as extracellular 'signallers', and can get 'stuck'. When your body's response to stress gets stuck or prolonged, your body can't heal at a cellular level, and symptoms and illness begin to arise.

Supporting my mitochondria, and removing the underlying infections, toxins, and pathogens that were affecting my health at a cellular level, finally helped me to resolve the adrenal dysfunction I had suffered from for so many years.

THE PRACTICAL STUFF

WHAT IS ADRENAL DYSFUNCTION?

Adrenal dysfunction (aka adrenal fatigue) is when your adrenal glands and HPA axis become depleted and dysregulated after a period of intense or prolonged stress or chronic illness and function below the necessary level.

This depletion results in symptoms such as a general feeling of being unwell, exhaustion, lowered immunity, and sleep disturbances, and in more serious cases, your adrenal function can be so diminished that you may be too exhausted to get out of bed for more than a few hours per day.

The great news is that you can support your adrenals to recover, and you can feel good again. It is important to note that recovery won't be overnight. It took time for your body to become so depleted, and sometimes it can be a slow journey to wellness, taking anywhere from six months to a couple of years.

HOW DID I GET IT?

Your adrenal glands are the small powerhouses that sit on top of each of your kidneys, and produce hormones such as your cortisol, estrogen, testosterone, and adrenaline. They modulate the way your body reacts to stress, as well as the way your tissues, organs, and glands function during stressful times.

If you have had an emotional stress, such as losing a loved one or the breakdown of a relationship, a physical stress such as a major illness, injury or surgery, environmental stress from toxins and chemicals, or any other constant, repeated, or intense stress, your adrenal glands can become fatigued. This is because they have been overstimulated and overproducing the hormones you needed to deal with these stresses, which has led to them becoming depleted, and to under-function.

WHAT ARE THE SYMPTOMS OF ADRENAL DYSFUNCTION?

You may be experiencing adrenal dysfunction if you regularly:

- feel tired for no reason, especially in the early morning and mid-afternoon
- don't wake feeling refreshed, even after a full night's sleep
- feel rundown or overwhelmed, and find it difficult to bounce back from stress or illness
- crave salty and/or sweet snacks
- feel more alert and energetic in the evening than you do all day.

THE IRIS FLASHLIGHT TEST - *AN INITIAL INDICATION ONLY*

(Source: Wilson James L. M.D. 2002, *Adrenal Fatigue: The 21st Century Stress Syndrome*, Smart Publications)

If you shine a flashlight across one of your eyes in a dark room, your pupil will adjust, and should remain smaller for one to two minutes if your adrenal glands are healthy. However, when your adrenal glands are under-functioning, your eye muscles become fatigued, and can't stay contracted.

After doing this at-home screening test, to have adrenal dysfunction properly diagnosed, please see a qualified medical practitioner (preferably one familiar with adrenal dysfunction) for a salivary DHEA/cortisol test. As well as getting an initial indication of adrenal dysfunction, this is also a good way to measure your progress as you rebuild your adrenals. It is best done at night, but a completely dark room will do.

HOW TO DO IT

You will need a small flashlight, a mirror, a dark room, and a timer.

1. Stand in front of a mirror in a dark room for at least 15 seconds and look straight ahead without blinking.
2. Hold the flashlight at eye level (about 8 inches away from your eye) and by the side of your head.

3. Slowly move the light until it is at a 45-degree angle to your
   iris. The light should not be pointing directly into your eye but
   should come in at an angle.
4. Hold the light steady and time how long your pupil can hold its
   contraction. Once it starts to 'pulse' or loses its contraction, stop
   the test.
5. Repeat on your other eye.

If your pupil dilates within the first 10-30 seconds, or begins to
quiver, but stays dilated for as long as 45 seconds before it contracts
again, adrenal dysfunction is indicated.

WHAT DO I DO IF I THINK I HAVE IT?

Find a good, integrative doctor

Finding the right practitioner wasn't easy, but played a key role in
my recovery. After asking around for recommendations for a good
doctor, I heard about integrative medicine for the first time. I will
always be grateful I was steered down this path early on.

Test, don't guess

Having a name for what was causing my symptoms meant that
they could be treated properly. For me, this meant testing my
hormone levels (salivary DHEA/cortisol, TSH, ACTH, thyroid,
and testosterone). I also did food sensitivity, and amino acid and

transmitter level testing to ascertain what imbalances I was suffering from, how they were affecting my body, and what supplements would be helpful.

Reduce your stress

I found that the two most effective ways I was able to reduce my stress levels were to adjust the expectations I had of myself, and to start saying no to the things that I did not have the capacity to do.

Make resting as much as possible a priority

When my doctor told me that to recover, I would need to rest as much as possible, I looked at her with scepticism. As the single mother of a five-year-old, how was I supposed to achieve this? I desperately needed to nap every day. When I didn't, I was exhausted, dizzy, overwhelmed and over emotional. My son got used to mummy's nap time, and our day was planned around this.

Learn to calm your overstimulated nervous system

I found that the best way to calm my nervous system was to find ways to still my mind. Although I found it very challenging at first, through closing my eyes listening to gentle, instrumental music and guided meditations, I was finally able to find that quiet place in my head and to slow my overactive thoughts.

Take supplements to help support and strengthen your body

The stress that led to depleted adrenal glands had also led me to my being deficient in many of the essential vitamins and minerals, nutrients, and hormones that my body needed to function effectively.

I found some supplements to be very helpful:

- Herbs played a big role in my recovery. In particular, ashwagandha, passionflower, Californian poppy, ziziphus, and Siberian ginseng helped me to support and strengthen my body.

- B5, B6 and B12 helped my energy levels, and more. B5 helps to produce the enzyme that contributes to cellular respiration and the breakdown of our fats, proteins, and carbohydrates. B6 acts in several of the pathways that are used to create our adrenal hormones, and B12 helps with energy production, cell repair, and the maintenance of our red blood cells.

- Vitamin C was an essential building block for the recovery of my adrenal glands. Buffered or liposomal vitamin C, in combination with bioflavonoids, are generally the best forms.

- Magnesium helped with my muscle cramps and improved my sleep.

- Bioidentical hormones helped with my low and unbalanced hormones.

The supplements I wish I had known about in 2008:

- MitoRestore helps support cellular renewal, maximise ATP production, and improve energy levels.
- BioActive Carbon Minerals support mitochondrial function.
- TUDCA Plus supports mitochondrial health and helps your liver metabolise high cortisol.

Please note that there are many other supplements that can be helpful. Your healthcare professionals may recommend other remedies, and you should follow their advice.

Understand that food is medicine, and you are what you eat

Over time, I learned what and how to eat to support my adrenals. Eating small nutrient-dense meals throughout the day and ensuring they each contained protein kept my energy levels more balanced. I stopped eating sugar; it gave me an immediate energy spike, but that spike was quickly followed a 'crash', tears, and feelings of low mood. Because of some digestive symptoms, I did a food sensitivity test, and found that avoiding those foods for three months while my gut healed from the inflammation, helped enormously.

Find something beautiful to appreciate each day

I found that there was enormous value in the simple act of noticing beauty around me. On the worst days, when I would switch my focus from how I felt, to the way the sun illuminated the trees, or the scent of a beautiful flower, it would bring my attention back to the fact that the world is beautiful.

Helpful resources

Dr. James Wilson was the first to coin the phrase 'adrenal fatigue' and is well-known for his book, Wilson James L. M.D. 2002, *Adrenal Fatigue: The 21st Century Stress Syndrome, Smart Publications*. This book is the culmination of Dr. Wilson's 24 years of clinical experience and research, and helps readers understand how stress affects your health, and determine if they have adrenal fatigue. Beginning with a diagnostic questionnaire, he explains the causes, symptoms, and how to treat it through lifestyle and dietary modification.

This comprehensive book contains many valuable insights, including the initial screening testing you can do at home. This book was a well-loved resource for me in the early days.

'YOU DON'T ALWAYS
HAVE TO BE GRATEFUL
THAT IT ISN'T WORSE.'

UNKNOWN

CHAPTER THREE

HEAVY METAL TOXICITY
WINNING THE LOTTERY

AFTER RECOVERING FROM ADRENAL DYSFUNCTION, FOR THREE YEARS I MOSTLY FELT GOOD AGAIN. IT WAS TRICKY BALANCING WORK WITH SPENDING AS MUCH TIME AS POSSIBLE WITH MY YOUNG SON, BUT I WAS HAPPY AND GENERALLY WELL. I WAS SLEEPING OK, MY BIOIDENTICAL HORMONES WERE KEEPING ME BALANCED, AND I WAS NO LONGER UNDERWEIGHT. MY SON AND I WERE ACTIVE, MOUNTAIN BIKING, HIKING, AND SURFING EVERY WEEKEND.

Although nervous about whether I was well enough yet, two years after being diagnosed with adrenal dysfunction, I began working again. Despite still feeling sad about losing my job at the Museum, I loved my new contract roles, first as Producer of the Melbourne Design Festival, then as the Curator of the Melbourne Design Awards. However, as a single mother, I needed the security of an ongoing position, and to ensure that I was as employable as possible.

Knowing that having digital experience would make me more marketable, I talked my way into a job at one of Australia's top three digital agencies. In my interview, I admitted that I had no experience in digital, but emphasised that I brought 20 years' project management experience and was a quick learner. They took me on, and over the next three years I gained knowledge in all aspects of the design, build, and maintenance of major websites. I loved it.

A sudden overnight return of adrenal dysfunction symptoms came as a shock and knocked me sideways. The severity of the symptoms was compounded by the trauma of being so sick a second time after believing that it would never happen again.

My stress threshold was normally very high. My colleagues had told me that calm is my superpower, and they enjoyed being on my project teams for that reason. I had just experienced a period of high stress, but it wasn't as severe as six years earlier, and I didn't dream it could affect me so dramatically. But it did. My weight plummeted to 47 kg, my hair came out in handfuls, crushing exhaustion and insomnia took hold, heart palpitations woke me at 4:00 am every day, and my hormone levels plummeted. Every meal caused digestive distress.

This time there were new symptoms too. My kidney function was reduced. My skin bruised simply with touch. My feet had fissures so deep that they cracked and bled when I stepped out of bed. My tongue was swollen and scalloped, and extreme fermentation in my intestinal system caused severe bloating, pain, and round-the-clock belching. My prolactin levels were ten times higher than they should be, and my nipples were burning. I could only get to sleep at night if I walked and belched for an hour first. My sleep was severely disrupted. For the first and only time in my life, I wasn't sure I could keep putting one foot in front of the other.

My doctor was mystified by my new symptoms and couldn't offer any new advice or treatment aside from it being another adrenal 'flare'. The other doctors and specialists I saw couldn't either. The experience of previously losing my job and my whole world almost crumbling was still very close to the surface. I felt lost and scared, and it was a very challenging time.

I heard about another integrative doctor, and fortunately, she was taking new patients. After talking through my health history, she asked if I had ever been tested for heavy metals. I didn't even know this could be a thing. A hair mineral analysis showed that I had problems detoxing, and that I had the highest levels of mercury and cadmium that she had ever seen.

I thought that I had won the lottery, and that fate had led me to my new doctor and what was causing my adrenal issues. Although I was facing another long slow treatment, I was confident that once I reduced the toxic heavy metal load, I would be well again.

Research into the source of heavy metal toxicity opened my eyes to the fact that heavy metals are everywhere around us in our everyday lives, and not being able to detox properly meant that over time I had accumulated high levels. Testing also showed low stomach acid, h pylori and gut dysbiosis, indicating that the heavy metals were affecting my digestive and immune systems. My doctor suggested slow and gentle chelation with liquid zeolites.

Although I struggled every day with the symptoms, I managed to keep working. I was barely getting enough sleep to function. The exhaustion was crushing, and there were many days when I wasn't sure how I would get through the day. I did though, and through the next day and the next. After two years of diligent treatment, my hair analysis tests showed a reduction in the levels of toxic metals. However, I still didn't feel much better, and was very discouraged.

I sought out an integrative doctor who had more experience in heavy metal and gut issues. Both a 6-hour urine DMSA challenge and an OligoScan (1) showed that my intracellular heavy metal levels were still very high. He explained that as you chelate the metals out of your body, the ones stored deeper in your tissues move into circulation, and that it is important to continue slowly removing them until the symptoms are gone. This can be a very long process when your levels are as high as mine.

Wondering how long my body could cope with the toxic burden, I was keen to get them out of my body as quickly as possible. However, I quickly learned that for people like me with very high toxin levels, genetic detox issues, and sulphur sensitivity, it is critical to go slowly when removing toxins. If you move metals out of your tissues too quickly and don't bind them properly, they can redistribute in new places such as in your brain, and cause dangerous symptoms. The larger the amount that you mobilise, and the more quickly, the more dramatic the symptoms can be.

Over the next few years, I tried a number of different binders, but it was when I finally got onto Microbe Formulas' treatment protocol that I made better progress in a couple of months than I had with any other treatment.

I now understand that as well as the specific binders I used to remove the heavy metals, the other vital factor in my success was using the approach I learned about from Dr. Todd Watts and Dr. Jay Davidson, the co-founders of Microbe Formulas. This included first supporting my detox pathways, immune system, and mitochondrial function so my body had the energy to enable the detox, then treating other infections, such as parasites, that were contributing to the issue, and finally, binding the heavy metals properly so they could be excreted safely. This approach is detailed later in this chapter.

THE PRACTICAL STUFF

WHAT ARE HEAVY METALS?

There are two types of heavy metals. Organic heavy metals are in a form that your body can use and are fundamental to your health, and inorganic heavy metals are in a form that your body can't use and can harm your health. Therefore, it is important that you have enough of the organic metals your body needs for its functions, and that you remove the inorganic metals that can cause disease, such as aluminium, mercury, cadmium, and lead.

Inorganic heavy metals are found all over the world in your air, food, water, and ground. They are in the things you use, consume, and are exposed to every day, such as anti-perspirants, aluminium foil, cans and cookware, tap water, dental fillings, tobacco smoke, rice, air pollution, auto exhaust, cosmetics, vaccines, and batteries. Over time, heavy metals can accumulate in your tissues without you even realizing that it is happening.

Heavy metal toxicity (aka heavy metal poisoning) can be behind digestive issues, brain fog, insomnia, autoimmune disease, and chronic health conditions, can result in damaged or reduced mental and central nervous function, and can damage vital organs — such as the liver, heart, endocrine glands, and kidneys.

WHAT ARE THE SYMPTOMS OF HEAVY METAL TOXICITY?

Common symptoms of heavy metal toxicity are:

- fatigue
- dizziness and light-headedness
- headaches
- digestion issues
- compromised ability to digest fats
- joint and muscle pain
- anxiety and depression
- irregular menstrual cycles
- infertility
- blood sugar imbalances
- numbness or tingling in your extremities
- insomnia or sleep disturbances
- night sweats.

Heavy metal toxicity is also known for producing symptoms that are often mistaken for chronic conditions, such as:

- chronic fatigue syndrome
- depression
- multiple sclerosis
- fibromyalgia

as well as many others.

It is important to note that symptoms can have multiple causes, for instance night sweats are common in Lyme patients with babesiosis. Dr. Richard Horowitz has put together a differential diagnostic table that will help you and your healthcare professionals get to the underlying aetiologies, as often there are more than one, and they need to be treated wholistically for you to fully recover. [2]

HOW CAN I TEST FOR HEAVY METALS?

There are many ways that people test for heavy metals, and each has its strengths and drawbacks. Common tests that are used include hair tissue mineral analysis (HTMA), provoked urine challenge, blood testing, OligoScan, and Quiksilver's Tri-test for mercury.

Heavy metal testing is challenging because:

- Test results depend on your body's capability to excrete metals. Most people who have heavy metal toxicity have a compromised ability to detox, so tests will only show anything if their levels are very high.

- Toxic metals will not always show up in your hair or urine, because they are often buried deep in your fat cells, liver, kidneys, and other areas of your body, and sometimes will only be revealed after you have been on a detox program for an extended period.

- Toxic metals are only found in high concentrations in your blood for a short period of time after an acute exposure because your body quickly moves the metals into places where they will do less damage. Most of us accumulate heavy metals through small exposures over a long period of time, so a blood test will not be accurate.

• Different metals are excreted in different ways, so one type of testing may miss metals that another one would pick up.

Your integrative doctor will have a preferred method of diagnosing/testing.

HOW DO I GET RID OF THEM?

Heavy metals do not leave your body easily or on their own, so you must remove them from your body and bloodstream by mobilising, binding, and eliminating them safely. The best way to do this is:

Supporting your drainage pathways

Opening your drainage pathways means ensuring that you are moving your bowels two or three times a day, and supporting your kidneys, liver, and lymphatic system to filter out the toxins.

If the pathways your body uses to eliminate toxins are not working well before you start detoxing or killing pathogens, it can lead to backups. These backups can cause unwanted symptoms like fatigue, joint pain, and brain fog and can make your body more toxic. There are many supplements that will help you support your drainage pathways, but I found that the best ones, formulated specifically for this task, are produced by Microbe Formulas. The 'Learn' section of their website includes many videos and articles on this subject, and you can find guidance on what to take, and how to take it, to support your drainage pathways.

Supporting your immune system and mitochondrial function so your body can deal with the mobilised toxins, and rebuild your damaged tissues and immune system

Most cells in your body contain mitochondria, which provide the energy for your body to carry out important functions like detoxification, signalling your immune system to fight any infections you have, and stimulating the death of damaged cells.

However, underlying issues you have such as viruses, parasites, heavy metals, medications, and severe oxidative stress can cause mitochondrial damage and dysfunction. This can result in low energy, the build-up of toxin levels, and a decline in your immune system health and the ability of your cells to repair. So, it is essential to support your mitochondrial energy to improve your energy, promote healing, and maintain your lasting health.

Supplements that helped me enormously in this regard are three of Microbe Formulas' products:

• MitoRestore supports your cellular energy levels, which helps with detox, the renewal of your cells, and immune support.

- Biomolecular Oxygen improves the oxygen levels in your tissues, which is important for the respiration of your cells, and for healing.

- BioActive Carbon Minerals provide the trace minerals and amino acids that will support detox through delivering your body what it needs to help produce your cellular energy.

Affectionately called 'the three amigos' by many people that use them, I can see myself taking all three of these supplements for the long term. Other helpful mitochondrial supplements I have heard about include Research Nutritionals' ATP360 and CoQ10 Power, and ENADA's NADH, L-carnitine.

Using fulvic acid and carbon-based binders to absorb and remove the toxins

Binders assist your body to reduce toxins and are a critical part of any detox protocol. Having tried most of the binders that are available, I found fulvic acid and carbon-based binders such as Microbe Formulas' BioActive Carbon BioTox, Foundation and MetChem to be game changers.

They are very effective in binding unwanted elements including everything from mycotoxins, herbicides, pesticides, mould, heavy metals, chemicals, and radioactive elements. (2)

They can be taken with food, will nourish rather than strip your microbiome (3), are safe long-term, and have high-energy carbon and oxygen that your cells need. You can take more than one of them at the same time, depending on which things you want to target. The Learn section on the Microbe Formulas website has articles and videos that will help you learn about these binders, which one to use for what issue, and how to take them.

As with any new supplements, it is important to start low and slow. If it seems that you cannot tolerate something, reduce the dose a lot to a tolerable level, and slowly build it up. Using this method, I was able to make good progress by working from sensitive dosing to aggressive dosing over time.

Other binders such as Biocidin's G.I. Detox can also be very effective.

Other ways to support your heavy metal detox:

- Follow an anti-inflammatory diet. You can find information about the paleo autoimmune diet that I followed (and recipes) on the Autoimmune Wellness website.

- Sweat it out in an infrared sauna. Far infrared saunas are one of the most effective methods of detoxing. The deep penetration of infrared heat releases toxins that have passed from the organs to the fat layers just beneath the skin, and they are eliminated in your perspiration.

Please note: There are things to consider, to ensure you use sauna therapy safely and effectively. For instance, regular saunas can deplete minerals from your body, and you have to be careful if you have some medical conditions, such as POTS with low blood pressure. It is important to research precautions, as well as pre and post session protocols, before embarking on sauna therapy

How to keep your heavy metals in a safe range after chelation:

• Use aluminium-free deodorant.

• Avoid cigarette smoke.

• Reduce shellfish and fish in your diet.

• Avoid unfiltered tap water.

• Reduce the arsenic in rice before eating it. To do this, thoroughly rinse the rice while it's raw. Then cook 1 cup of rice in 6 cups of water. Cover the pot while it's cooking, as the more water that stays in the pot, the better. When the rice is fully cooked, strain it. Preparing rice this way can reduce arsenic by up to 45%, and works best with long-grain and basmati rice.

THE PITFALLS OF DETOX

There are many pitfalls in heavy metal detoxification, and I fell into most of them.

In summary, I learned that:

• It took many years to accumulate the metals; you cannot expect to remove them quickly, and to do so is dangerous.

- It is important to work with a practitioner who is trained in proper heavy metal chelation protocols. When heavy metal detox is done correctly and safely, you can recover from unexplained illnesses.

- To successfully chelate heavy metals out of your body and brain, and to prevent the dangers of re-absorption, you must use a true 'chelator'. Things like cilantro or chlorella don't have the molecular structure to permanently bind to the heavy metals so they can be removed from your body through your bowel movements and urine. Binding them permanently ensures they are not reabsorbed into your bloodstream.

- When a chelating agent moves out of your body, it takes heavy metals with it, leaving a lower concentration area behind. This causes the metals that are stored deeper in the body to be stirred up, move out of your tissues into circulation, and be redistributed somewhere else. This sometimes causes further damage and an increase in symptoms.

- It is essential to first prepare your detoxification pathways such as your liver, kidneys, lymphatic, and intestinal systems.

- As well as exhausting your detoxification pathways, which allows the accumulation of other toxins, heavy metals can cause other issues by providing a haven for pathogens such as candida and Lyme. Your immune cells will not come near toxic metals, so these pathogens are able to adapt and hide from your immune system by staying near the metals. Many Lyme disease sufferers have heavy metal issues, and therefore both need to be addressed to achieve lasting recovery.

- Raising glutathione in your cells can help move heavy metals
  out of your deeper cellular stores. Because I can't tolerate oral
  glutathione due to its sulphur content, I use riboceine to increase
  my glutathione levels. I also do coffee enemas, which are thought
  to enhance your body's detoxification system. (5) Other things
  that can drive glutathione production are NAC, and Continual-G
  (available online).

- As well as removing the heavy metals that have built up in your
  body, you need to reduce or remove the source(s) of your exposure
  to heavy metals to ensure your long-term health.

Raising glutathione in your cells can help move heavy metals out of
your deeper cellular stores. Because I can't tolerate oral glutathione
due to its sulphur content, I use riboceine to increase my glutathione
levels. I also do coffee enemas, which are thought to enhance
your body's detoxification system. (5) Other things that can drive
glutathione production are NAC, and Continual-G (available online).

HELPFUL REFERENCES AND RESOURCES

(1) The OligoScan is discussed in Jon Gamble's latest book, which also
contains case studies and comparisons. - Gamble, J 2022, *Mastering
Chronic Disease: Toxicity, Deficiency and Infection*, Karuna Publishing,
Woolongong, NSW, Australia

Because the use of spectrophotometry to assay minerals is a new
method, Lumometrix has sponsored several clinical trials to gain

insight from some experts in the field. These clinical trials are documented in the following article: Gamble, Jon v17 2022, Clinical Evaluation Report for OligoScan Spectrophotometry, Yerinbool, NSW, Australia

For more information on the OligoScan, and scientific references, go to www.oligoscan.co.nz

(2) Dr. Horowitz's Sixteen-Point Differential Diagnosis MSIDS Map can be found in his book, Horowitz, Richard I M.D. 2017, *How Can I Get Better? An Action Plan for Treating Resistant Lyme and Chronic Disease*, St. Martin's Griffin, New York, New York, p 50-65

(3) https://microbeformulas.com/blogs/microbe-formulas/9-old-school-toxin-binders-plus-meet-a-better-binder - 9 Old-School Toxin Binders (Plus, Meet a Better Binder) - Microbe Formulas™https://microbeformulas.com/blogs/microbe-formulas/10-reasons-why-you-need-carbon-based-binders

https://pubmed.ncbi.nlm.nih.gov/12663188

Bäckström M, Dario M, Karlsson S, Allard B. Effects of a fulvic acid on the adsorption of mercury and cadmium on goethite. Sci Total Environ. 2003 Mar 20;304(1-3):257-68. doi: 10.1016/S0048-9697(02)00573-9. PMID: 12663188.

https://pubmed.ncbi.nlm.nih.gov/15092099

Lafrance P, Villeneuve JP, Mazet M, Ayele J, Fabre B. Organic compounds adsorption onto activated carbon: the effect of association between dissolved humic substances and pesticides. Environ Pollut.

1991;72(4):331-44. doi: 10.1016/0269-7491(91)90006-i. PMID: 15092099.

https://pubmed.ncbi.nlm.nih.gov/28233210

Pozdnyakov IP, Sherin PS, Salomatova VA, Parkhats MV, Grivin VP, Dzhagarov BM, Bazhin NM, Plyusnin VF. Photooxidation of herbicide amitrole in the presence of fulvic acid. Environ Sci Pollut Res Int. 2018 Jul;25(21):20320-20327. doi: 10.1007/s11356-017-8580-x. Epub 2017 Feb 23. PMID: 28233210.

(4) https://pubmed.ncbi.nlm.nih.gov/28223733

Swidsinski A, Dörffel Y, Loening-Baucke V, Gille C, Reißhauer A, Göktas O, Krüger M, Neuhaus J, Schrödl W. Impact of humic acids on the colonic microbiome in healthy volunteers. World J Gastroenterol. 2017 Feb 7;23(5):885-890. doi: 10.3748/wjg.v23. i5.885. PMID: 28223733; PMCID: PMC5296205.

(5) Lam, L.K.T, Sparnins, V.L., Wattenburg, L.W., 1982. Cancer Research, 42:1193-1198, 1982. "Isolation and Identification of Kahweal Palmitate and Cafestol Palmitate as Active Constituents of Green Coffee Beans That Enhances Gluathione S-transferase activity in the Mouse."

www.klinghardtacademy.com

Dr. Deitrich Klinghardt, MD, PhD, pioneered many diagnostic and detoxification strategies for the chemical and heavy metal toxicity that is at the core of many medical issues. His website is full of helpful resources, and I also found his YouTube videos provided valuable information.

www.myersdetox.com

Wendy Myers, FDN, founded myersdetox.com to communicate her expert knowledge and research on heavy metal toxicity, detoxification, supplements, and nutrition. I found her website and podcasts to be a wealth of information about heavy metal toxicity.

www.quicksilverscientific.com

Dr. Chris Shade is a globally recognized expert on mercury, heavy metals, and the body's detoxification system. I spent hours watching his YouTube videos and listening to him speak in podcasts and learned much in the process.

www.microbeformulas.com

The Microbe Formulas website is my all-time favourite health resource for information on heavy metal toxicity, mould illness, parasites, Lyme disease and co-infections. On their site, Dr. Todd Watts and Dr. Jay Davidson of Microbe Formulas provide numerous videos and articles. You can search the Learn section by topic and find informative and enlightening resource materials as well as effective treatment and maintenance protocol advice. The support team at Microbe Formulas are fantastic. I called them many times to ask numerous questions about their products and treatment protocols, and I can't recommend them highly enough.

'NEVER LET THE
THINGS YOU CANNOT
DO PREVENT YOU
FROM DOING WHAT
YOU CAN.'

COACH JOHN WOODEN

SMALL INTESTINE BACTERIAL OVERGROWTH (SIBO)
THINGS OVERGROWING IN THE WRONG PLACE

IN 2015, SMALL INTESTINAL BACTERIAL OVERGROWTH (SIBO) WAS NOT SOMETHING GENERAL PRACTITIONERS IN AUSTRALIA WERE FAMILIAR WITH YET. WHEN I STARTED ASKING QUESTIONS ABOUT IT, BOTH MY DOCTOR AND A GASTROENTEROLOGIST SAID THAT IT DIDN'T EXIST, THAT IT WAS SOMETHING THAT HAD BEEN 'INVENTED' BY NATUROPATHS.

WHEN I DESCRIBED VOMITING AIR FOR 20 MINUTES IN THE SHOWER EVERY MORNING FROM GUT FERMENTATION, THE GASTROENTEROLOGIST I HAD WAITED MONTHS TO SEE TOLD ME THAT MY UPPER AND LOWER GI WERE NORMAL, AND THAT I WAS 'JUST SWALLOWING TOO MUCH AIR WHEN I ATE'.

When my heavy metal toxicity was diagnosed, the most distressing symptoms I had were digestive. I had round-the-clock belching, abdominal pain and bloating, constipation, and sensitivity to any food with a starch or carb content.

I'd had intermittent digestive issues on and off through my life. My symptoms had always been given that mysterious and all-encompassing term Irritable Bowel Syndrome (IBS), with no suggested treatment except to avoid the problem foods. This time however, the symptoms were extreme and relentless.

From what I had read, SIBO was a likely candidate, as my symptoms were mainly in my upper GI. As my doctor didn't specialise in gut issues, I needed to find someone with expertise in diagnosing and treating SIBO. My search led me to a wonderful naturopath, who diagnosed methane dominant SIBO through a lactulose and glucose breath test.

I embarked on a journey that spanned many years and strategies, but five years later, I was still bloated, constipated, and belching around the clock, and having to go for extensive walks daily to relieve the pain and be able to sleep. Over that time span, I had tried every available treatment including antibiotics, herbal antibiotics, antivirals, antimicrobials, the elemental diet, and the SIBO diet. I waited two years to consult with the best-known gut naturopath in the world, but after a year on his special tonic I still had symptoms. During this time, my diet continued to be extremely limited to what I could tolerate – only meat and vegetables.

Over time, I learned that there is always an underlying reason that SIBO initially develops. When you have SIBO, or any other digestive issue (such as candida), it is because your body has changed internally in response to its environment.

I believe my SIBO started after having shigellosis, a bacterial infection known to damage the migrating motor complex. Because my migrating motor complex was compromised, bacteria was not being cleared from my small intestine into my large intestine between meals and during fasting at night. As well as having shigellosis, I already had a compromised terrain due to the high levels of toxins and pathogens I had been carrying – for instance issues with G.I. motility is often seen with Lyme disease and dysautonomia of the digestive tract

There are many reasons that SIBO doesn't resolve after the standard treatment of a low FODMAP diet combined with antimicrobial treatment. Your gut will only heal when you also clear the other culprits including parasites, infections, toxins, and heavy metals. It is important to note that it will take time for the environment of your gut to change and heal, but it will.

I was finally able to get on top of my long-term digestive issues when I cleared not only the bacteria, but also the toxins, pathogens, and infections that were affecting my terrain. It was amazing after all those years to finally be able to eat a wider variety of foods, and no longer to have the symptoms I had for so long.

Over the many years it took me to beat it, I learned some key things, outlined below, that might help you better understand this condition and your symptoms, as well as what might help assist in your long-term recovery.

THE PRACTICAL STUFF

WHAT IS SIBO?

SIBO is an overgrowth of bacteria that normally live in your gastrointestinal tract but have overgrown abnormally in your small intestine, a location not meant for so many bacteria.

The bacteria can:

- interfere with the normal digestion and absorption of your food and can damage the lining or membrane of your small intestine. This can lead to larger food particles not being fully digested, then entering your body and causing your immune system to react, as well as creating food allergies and/or sensitivities
- consume some of your food which can lead to deficiencies over time, such as in iron and B12, causing anaemia or chronic low ferritin
- consume the food which you can't absorb due to damage to the lining of your small intestine, which can lead to a vicious cycle of continual overgrowth
- produce gas in your small intestine after consuming your food. This gas can cause abdominal bloating, abdominal pain, constipation, diarrhea (or both), belching, and flatulence
- deconjugate your bile, which decreases proper fat absorption, and

can lead to deficiencies of vitamins A & D, as well as fatty stools

- enter your bloodstream, causing immune system reactions, chronic fatigue, body pain, and burden on your liver
- excrete acids which can lead to neurological and cognitive symptoms.

SIBO is generally categorised into two different types, differentiated by the main type of gas produced by the bacterial overgrowth in your intestines. Each type is unique and requires a different treatment approach.

Hydrogen dominant (SIBO – D)

If you have SIBO with diarrhea, you likely have an overgrowth of hydrogen-producing bacteria. The bacteria produce the hydrogen gas as a by-product of fermenting carbohydrates in your digestive system. This is a normal process that normally occurs in your large intestine. When bacteria colonise your small intestine and produce hydrogen gas in large amounts, it can cause fast transit time and loose stools.

Hydrogen – sulphide dominant

Our bodies use sulphur for detoxing, and convert small amounts into hydrogen sulphide. If too much hydrogen sulphide is produced, it can cause SIBO.

OTHER TYPES OF SMALL INTESTINAL OVERGROWTH

Small intestinal methanogen overgrowth (SIMO)

Although hydrogen production can come from a wide variety of bacteria, methane production is limited to only a few, known as methanogens. They are technically not bacteria, but single-cell organisms that feed off the hydrogen produced by bacteria, and produce methane as a by-product. Methane dominant SIBO is associated with constipation and slower transit time. When there is methane production, there must be hydrogen-producing bacteria as well, and they both must be treated.

Small intestinal fungal overgrowth (SIFO)

Sometimes fungal overgrowth can occur in the small intestine as well. This is common in people with SIBO, and must be treated with anti-fungals for them to recover fully.

HOW DO I KNOW IF I HAVE SIBO?

The small intestine is a hard place to get to, so there is no perfect test. An endoscopy only reaches the top part, a colonoscopy only reaches the bottom, and the middle portion (over five metres, or around 17 feet) is not easily accessible, so it is difficult to get a sample to culture. Stool testing predominantly reflects the large intestine.

The trio-smart™ breath test measures the levels of hydrogen, methane, and hydrogen sulphide in your breath over a couple of hours after

lactulose or glucose consumption, and is the best way to get a
complete picture of any overgrowth.

WHY DO I HAVE IT, AND HOW CAN I PREVENT RELAPSE?

I learned that with SIBO, it is essential not only to treat the
symptoms, but also to identify and treat the underlying causes.
The bacteria can repopulate the small intestine within two weeks
of finishing treatment, so these causes must still be addressed for
lasting recovery.

THESE UNDERLYING CAUSES CAN BE:

Parasites, heavy metal toxicity, or Lyme disease

Chronic SIBO may be caused by the impact of parasites, heavy
metal toxicity, or Lyme disease on your immune system, or through
affecting the nervous system in your gut.

Nerve damage from previous food poisoning

The migrating motor complex propels bacteria from your small
intestine into your large intestine between meals and during fasting
at night. Food poisoning can damage the migrating motor complex.

Anatomical/structural alteration effecting the small intestine

Structural issues such as adhesions, obstructions, blind loops, or
ileocecal valve issues can impede the clearance of bacteria. This

allows bacteria to be trapped, or causes the backflow of bacteria into your small intestine from your large intestine.

REASONS YOUR PROTECTIVE ANTIBACTERIAL MECHANISMS ARE NOT WORKING

Low stomach acid

A healthy stomach is acidic and kills off the microbes that are present in your food. However, many things can lead to achlorhydria and therefore to SIBO, such as the use of proton pump inhibitors.

Pancreatic insufficiency

Reduced function of the pancreas and its antibacterial proteolytic enzymes can lead to bacterial overgrowth.

Immunodeficiency syndromes

Conditions such as IgA deficiencies can predispose people to mucosal infections, atopy, and even autoimmune issues.

Motility disorders

Some conditions can cause poor flow through the small intestine and lead to SIBO. Some of these are:

- Lyme disease
- scleroderma
- autonomic neuropathy
- post-radiation enteropathy

- vagal nerve dysfunction
- migrating motor complex dysfunction.

Healing, and to prevent relapse

Resolving your gut issues requires getting to the root of the problem. To do this, in addition to killing off the bacteria or methanogens, you need to:

- boost your drainage so that your body can cope with detox
- kill off the parasites (yes, we all have them) and other chronic infections
- remove toxins
- pay attention to what you eat
- move your body to bolster your immune system and drain your body's lymph.

As well as the antimicrobials and anti-parasitic herbs that you take, BioActive Carbon, liver-supportive herbs, TUDCA Plus, and lymph-supportive herbs can all help.

It is important to note that gas and bloating can also be due to many other reasons, such as candida overgrowth in the lower intestine, food intolerances, and allergies.

WHAT IS DIE-OFF?

'Die-off' reactions (also known as 'Jarisch-Herxheimer reactions' or 'a herx') occur when infections such as bacteria, parasites, or fungi are killed off rapidly without your body's elimination organs being able to keep up with their removal. As the bugs die, your body can become overwhelmed with the toxins and proteins they release. This can lead to inflammation, and can present as fever and chills, muscle aches, fatigue, brain fog, rashes, headaches, or a worsening of your normal symptoms (such as abdominal pain and bloating, diarrhea, or constipation).

Sometimes it is hard to tell if you are having a die-off reaction, a flare of your symptoms, or a new infection. You may not be tolerating the treatment, or you may be reacting to a different food or supplement. Sometimes these things can happen at the same time. The main difference is that die-off is temporary, and it usually starts within a few days or a week after you start a new treatment and ends within a few days or a week.

For this reason, it is handy to keep notes when you make any changes to your protocol, like starting a new antimicrobial or antifungal treatment, or making changes to your diet. This can make it easier to link the timing of the new symptoms with any changes, so you can more easily determine what is a die-off and what is a reaction caused by something else.

What can I do to minimise die-off symptoms?

Effective things you can do to minimise your die-off symptoms are the same as when removing heavy metals:

- Prepare your elimination pathways.
- Support your immune system and mitochondrial function so your

body can deal with the mobilised toxins and rebuild your damaged tissues and immune system.

- Use fulvic acid and carbon-based binders to absorb and remove the toxins.

You can also:

- Alkalizing your body with sodium bicarbonate or tri salts, and using up to 2000 mg of glutathione for die-off reactions, as recommended by Dr. Horowitz. (1)
- Reduce your dose and build up to a full dose more slowly.
- Stay hydrated.
- Rest as much as possible.
- Take Epsom salt baths.
- Sweat it out in a sauna.

It helps to include antioxidants in your protocol, to help your body deal with the effects of the inflammation.

WHAT ARE MY TREATMENT OPTIONS?

SIBO Diet

Changing your diet can dramatically reduce your symptoms and is often an important part of any treatment protocol. Bacteria mainly feed on carbohydrates (except insoluble fibre), so most diets that people use for SIBO reduce the fermentable carbohydrates. Limiting the bacteria's food supply helps reduce the number of bacteria, which then will reduce your digestive symptoms. The goal is to feed you, not the bacteria, and to have the least restrictive diet that helps you manage your symptoms.

The main diets people use are:

• the SIBO diet

• SCD

• low FODMAP

• Cedars Sinai Low Fermentation.

Pharmaceutical antibiotics

Antibiotics are one of the quickest and most effective treatment options when you are suffering from SIBO. They work by either killing the bacteria in the small intestine or by stopping them from replicating. The main pharmaceutical antibiotics used for SIBO are Rifaximin (Xifaxan) and Neomycin. They are almost completely non-absorbable, which means they act only where they are needed locally in your intestines and don't cause systemic side effects. Metronidazole, a systemic antibiotic, is also sometimes used.

Herbal antibiotics

It doesn't matter whether antibiotics are made synthetically in a lab or are extracted from plants. Like pharmaceutical antibiotics, herbal antibiotics have also been found to be effective (2). One

of the benefits of herbs is that they can be combined to produce
a synergistic effect on the bacteria, therefore reducing the risk of
resistance. These combination formulas can be very effective, but
they can make it more challenging to know which herb has caused
an issue if you have an adverse reaction.

Many different herbs have antibiotic properties, but it is important
to find the right match and dose for you. It is best to be guided by
your medical practitioner. Some of the different herbs that can be
used to treat SIBO are listed below. I used every one of these:

- Allimed
- oregano oil
- berberine
- Neem Plus
- cinnamon
- pomegranate husk
- clove
- thyme
- Atrantil

Others such as Metagenics' Candibactin AR and Candibactin
BR have been published in the medical literature for treatment of
SIBO. There is also published medical literature on the helpfulness
of immunoglobulins from bovine source and spore base probiotics,
such as Mega IgG and MegaSporeBiotic.

Elemental diet

The elemental diet is used to treat SIBO by feeding you while starving the bacteria through replacing your meals for two to three weeks with powdered, pre-digested nutrients containing amino acids, carbohydrates, fats, vitamins, and minerals that absorb very quickly in the top of your GI. You can buy it pre-made or you can purchase ingredients online and make your own at home.

The elemental works quickly, is easy to purchase or make, and is very effective, reducing the need to do multiple rounds of antibiotics or antimicrobials. It can be expensive to buy though, and challenging to not eat solid foods for the time that you are on it. To give you enough calories, it is often high in sugars, which can lead to yeast overgrowth, so it can be helpful to take an anti-fungal while using the elemental diet.

WHAT IS A PROKINETIC AND WHY IS IT IMPORTANT?

Motility is everything.

Motility is the movement of food and waste through your intestinal tract and out of your body as stool. The wave-like movements of your migrating motor complex (MMC) push undigested food and waste, including excess bacteria, out of your small intestine and into your large intestine, where it can be excreted. If your MMC is not functioning properly, your food sits in the small intestine longer than it should, creating the perfect environment for bacterial or fungal overgrowth.

Prokinetics help promote movement through regulating the nerves of your small intestine. Taking a pharmaceutical or natural prokinetic at bedtime will make sure that the waste in your small intestine is being flushed out each night and bacteria does not build up.

Another important aspect of restoring your MMC function is to allow time for it to work. As the MMC's cleaning waves normally happen every 90 - 120 minutes when your stomach is empty, and take up to two hours to complete, to allow the MMC to work properly you need to wait four or more hours between meals and snacks, as any calories between meals (even water) will stop this function. Fasting for at least twelve hours at night is helpful too. Your MMC slows down at night, so the longer you can comfortably extend your fast, the better it can do its work.

Many practitioners suggest using a prokinetic to improve the movement and function of your gut for at least three to six months after SIBO treatment even if food poisoning is not behind your SIBO.

I take .5mg of prucalopride every night at bedtime. Dr. Mark Pimental, gastroenterology specialist, Associate Professor of medicine at Cedars-Sinai Medical Center and leading expert on SIBO, recommends this as the top prokinetic when taken in small doses at night, preferably on an empty stomach. Work with your health professional to determine which prokinetic is best for you. There are many pharmaceutical and natural options to choose from.

Magnesium deficiency can also affect gut motility, so have your serum and red blood cell magnesium levels checked. If you are deficient, taking extra magnesium can be helpful.

HELPFUL REFERENCES AND RESOURCES

(1) Horowitz, Richard I M.D. 2017, *How Can I Get Better? An Action Plan for Treating Resistant Lyme and Chronic Disease*, St. Martin's Griffin, New York, New York, p 382

(2) Chedid V, Dhalla S, Clarke JO, et al. Herbal therapy is equivalent to rifaximin for the treatment of small intestinal bacterial overgrowth. Glob Adv Health Med. 2014;3(3):16-24. doi:10.7453/gahmj.2014.019

www.siboinfo.com

This is a fantastic resource, with information and news about SIBO and its treatment by Dr. Allison Siebecker, ND, MSOM, LAc, who was the co-founder and former medical director of the SIBO Center for Digestive Health at The National University of Natural Medicine Clinic and has specialized in the treatment of SIBO since 2010.

www.sibosurvivor.com

This is a wonderful website with extensive information about SIBO, treatment, diet, and recipes. It provides links to where you can purchase SIBO-recommended products such as herbal antibiotics, elemental diet products, probiotics, and prokinetics. It was put together by a talented and informed content team of medical doctors, registered dieticians, naturopathic doctors, researchers, herbalists, and patients who have lived with IBS and SIBO.

www.thesibodoctor.com

The SIBO Doctor was founded by Dr. Nirala Jacobi, an internationally recognised expert in SIBO and other functional digestive disorders. Her website provides online courses for both patients and practitioners to learn about successful methods for treating SIBO, and lists a wide range of useful resources.

www.thehealthygut.com

Rebecca Coomes is the author of the world's first SIBO cookbooks, is the host of the SIBO Cooking Show, and hosts the SIBO podcast. Rebecca coaches SIBO patients through a 5-step method she has developed, she holds gut-health workshops, is a speaker on gut health and SIBO, and is a guest contributor and blogger on health and wellness sites.

'DON'T CONFUSE
MY BAD DAYS WITH
WEAKNESS. THOSE
ARE ACTUALLY THE
DAYS I AM FIGHTING
THE HARDEST.'

UNKNOWN

CHAPTER FIVE

BIOTOXIN ILLNESS
THE CURSE OF LIVING NEAR THE BEACH

I WILL NEVER FORGET WHEN MY DOCTOR ASKED ME IF I HAD BEEN EXPOSED TO MOULD, BECAUSE IT SEEMED LIKE SUCH AN ODD QUESTION AT THE TIME. BEING AN OUTDOORSY, NATURE-LOVING KIND OF GAL, I HAD NO IDEA MOULD COULD BE DANGEROUS, IT WAS JUST A FUNGUS, WASN'T IT?

When we moved into a new apartment the year before, I had noticed mould in the bathroom. But I was so happy to be living near the beach, having to clean a bit of mould off the shower didn't even register as inconvenient, much less hazardous. Little did I know.

At the time he asked, testing showed that my heavy metal levels were still very high after two years of treatment. I had been suffering from a worsening of the usual symptoms, but also had started experiencing new ones over the past year.

Along with the usual difficulty gaining weight, digestive distress, and insomnia, I had started to pee all the time. By all the time, I mean every half-hour around the clock, and in giant volume. My kidneys were not consolidating my urine properly, and this meant that I was lucky to get four to six hours of broken rest in any one night.

Exhaustion descended like a thick fog. I started reacting to more foods, and even the number of different vegetables I could tolerate had reduced. I was experiencing static shocks when I got dressed, brushed my hair, or touched metal objects, and the fermentation in my intestines was worse than ever before.

We had moved a year earlier to a lovely, modern apartment near the beach. It was tiny, but this was offset by its location. My son had been attending a fantastic school in the area for a year, and the decision to move nearby was an easy one. It was a great opportunity to live near his school, friends, and the beach. One of the best junior riders in the country, my son loved kiteboarding, and now could kite close to home at one of our city's best spots. For me, the draw of slow beach walks and lazy ocean swims was alluring. It would be the perfect place to recover from my heavy metal toxicity.

However, the decision to move collided with applying for a new job. I had been aware for a while that I needed to earn more money to afford the appointments and supplements that were helping me manage my symptoms. I had already re-mortgaged my apartment a couple of times, my credit card was maxxed out, and the situation was not sustainable.

When an opportunity to apply for a new job presented itself, I had to go for it. I knew that moving and applying for a new job at the same time would be stressful, but I just hoped that any bump in my recovery would be short-lived and worth it.

I spent weeks preparing for the interview. From the position description it sounded like it would utilise all the skills and experience I had gained so far, and was perfect for me. The interview went very well, and I began my new job shortly after we moved.

Exactly two weeks after we slept in the new apartment for the first time, and just as I started my new job, new symptoms came out of nowhere and knocked me sideways. I thought it was the stress-related 'flare' that I had anticipated, and that it would just take me a few weeks or months at the most to recover. But instead of getting better, my health continued to deteriorate over the rest of the year.

I battled through, month after month, too tired to even walk one block to the beach many days, but believing that the symptoms would settle in time. Finally, I booked in to see my doctor, and sobbed through the entire appointment.

Fortunately, he was 'mould-literate', and recognised some of my symptoms. After a quick Visual Contrast Sensitivity screening test confirmed his suspicions, he diagnosed me with biotoxin illness. In addition, through a nasal swab, he found that I had MARCoNS (Multiple Antibiotic Resistant Coagulase Negative), an antibiotic resistant staph infection residing deep in my nasal passages that affects 80% of people suffering from mould illness.

Once again, I stacked a diagnosis on top of the previous ones. I felt again that I'd had a major victory. Having learned that mould illness blocks up your detox pathways, perhaps this was the reason I had developed such high levels of heavy metals, and the heavy metals were behind my adrenal 'flares', right? Everything made sense, and hearing that the mould illness was treatable, I high fived my doctor, and whooped out loud. Once again, there was a light at the end of the tunnel.

I went home, looked around, and found mould everywhere. It was growing inside the door seal of my front-loading washing machine, behind the bulkheads in my bedroom, along the tops of the venetian blinds, behind the mixer in the shower, in the u-bends in the pipes beneath the kitchen and bathroom sinks, along the aluminium balcony door sills, inside the bathroom exhaust fan, and in the filters of the air conditioning unit. I loved long hot baths and showers, and it appeared that the mould did too. The black grout and dark brown tiles had helped disguise the extent of the problem in the shower. I felt the walls closing at the reality of my unhealthy environment.

Located in a modern building, the apartment was designed to maximise profit for the developers, not air flow for residents. My son's bedroom was legally classified as a 'study' and along with the bathroom, had no windows. Being close to the beach, the humidity was high and ventilation was inadequate, providing the perfect environment to nurture condensation and mould growth.

Thus began my education in and treatment for what I now understand is a widespread problem. Healing from mould toxicity requires safely removing the source of the mould, and detoxing your body. I prepared to move for the second time in as many years. Only blocks away, and still near the beach, the building was newer and better maintained. My son's room had big windows, and the apartment was mould-free. The long journey of recovery began.

THE KEY THINGS I LEARNED ALONG THE WAY:

Mould does not need to be visible to cause harm

I know someone who became very ill while living in an apartment two stories above an apartment that had been deemed uninhabitable due to mould. There was no visible mould in her own home. Mould spreads via spores, which are invisible and are carried through the air.

You won't get well in the same environment you got sick in

My doctor made it clear that we had to get out of that environment, that the first and most important step in healing would be to remove the source. No amount of detox could heal my body if I was still being exposed regularly to the source of the toxins. He explained that getting rid of mould is not always possible, and that even the most experienced remediation company might not be able to get rid of it entirely. When building materials are very porous (like plasterboard), the infestation can be so deep that no amount of excavation, cleaning, and fogging will entirely eradicate the issue. Sometimes it is better to move and start fresh.

You need to reduce the biotoxins

As with SIBO and heavy metals, you need to detox the things that are making you unwell. To remove the biotoxins that had accumulated in my body, my doctor recommended that I use a binder to attract and bind the toxins to facilitate their passage out of my body through my gastrointestinal tract.

Our most important detox organ, the liver, expels toxins into our bile, a digestive fluid that flows from our liver into our small intestines. Binders attach to biotoxins, heavy metals, and chemicals, escort them through our digestive tract, and stop them being reabsorbed before they are excreted. Removing toxins in this way, through the bowels, reduces the stress placed on the kidneys.

The journey to wellness is not easy, but it is possible

Recovery from biotoxin illness is not a quick process. I learned that, despite my best wishes, there was no magic pill and recovery was going to take a year or more. I realised the need to pace myself, and treat it as a marathon, not a sprint.

You may need to treat co-infections and other toxins

Because biotoxin illness can suppress your immune system, having it meant I was susceptible to contracting or reactivating other illnesses and pathogens such as Epstein Barr Virus or Lyme disease. In addition, as mould illness can block detox pathways, I needed to continue to treat my heavy metal toxicity.

Sometimes you need to get rid of everything

Mould spores can find their way into everything from books, to bedding, clothes, and furniture. Taking beds, furniture, and other objects from a mouldy home into a new home might mean that you bring those spores with you.

I have heard it said that when you have biotoxin illness, when you move, you should only take your drivers' licence with you. While this seems extreme, after the first year of treatment, I realised that the only way to stop exposing myself to mould spores would be to get rid of all the things from my previous home that could not be washed, like books, paintings, and soft furnishings like rugs.

THE PRACTICAL STUFF

WHAT IS MOULD ILLNESS?

Mould illness is a biotoxin illness, also known as chronic inflammatory response syndrome (CIRS), causing severe inflammation, and a cascade of other health effects.

Biotoxins are toxins produced by living organisms such as mould and bacteria. Biotoxin illness produces multiple symptoms across many of your body's systems at the same time, making it difficult to recognise as it mimics so many other illnesses. People have been misdiagnosed with other illnesses such as chronic fatigue, fibromyalgia, chronic sinus infections, depression, stress, allergies, PTSD, MS, dementia, IBS, ADD and more.

The key trigger is current or past exposure to biotoxins. Usually, this is an exposure to a water-damaged building, but there are other sources too, including tick bites, contaminated water, contaminated fish, or spider bites. Lyme disease and Babesia are both key triggers for CIRS.

Many people will become ill when exposed to high levels of biotoxins, but when they are removed from the exposure, most will recover through their body's detox mechanisms. However, around 25% of the population have a genetic variation that prevents them from being able to eliminate the biotoxins, triggering an inflammatory response. These people are at higher risk of developing biotoxin illness. How badly you are affected depends on your genetics and function of your detox system, total toxic load, and level of toxins you are exposed to. People in the same family can be affected in very different ways and experience very different symptoms.

Unfortunately, exposure to water-damaged buildings is very common, as around 40-50% of homes and commercial buildings have had water damage. It only takes 48 hours for dampness from a minor leak or water intrusion for mould, mould fragments, bacteria, and toxic mould by-products to develop on carpet, drywall, furniture, and other porous surfaces.

Mould also thrives in humid, moist air and in warm, dark places such as under refrigerators and inside washing machine door seals. It feeds on wood, paper, and organic materials and can grow in high-humidity environments in as little as 48-72 hours. It never grows alone. Bacteria are always present too, and together they release toxins and inflammagens that work synergistically to make you very ill.

Healing from mould toxicity requires safely removing the source of the mould, detoxing your body, as well as removing other sources of toxicity from your home, workplace, and other places that you spend time. Although it is overwhelming, you can recover.

It is important to note that having biotoxin or mould illness is different from having a fungal illness such as candida, or a mould or pollen allergy.

WHAT ARE THE COMMON SYMPTOMS?

One of the key features of biotoxin illness is that it causes multiple symptoms across many of the body's systems at the same time.

The most common symptoms are fatigue, memory and concentration issues, and inflammation and pain in almost any part of the body, but there are often widespread metabolic effects. The 37 most common symptoms are gathered into 13 clusters for the purpose of diagnosis.

If you have just one or two of the common symptoms and only in one cluster, it is unlikely that you have CIRS. It usually involves symptoms from at least six and up to ten symptom clusters. I had multiple symptoms in every one of the clusters.

It is important to note that symptoms can have multiple causes. Dr. Richard Horowitz has put together a differential diagnostic table that helps patients and their healthcare professionals get to the underlying aetiologies, as often there are more than one. (1)

Biotoxin illness (CIRS) symptom clusters

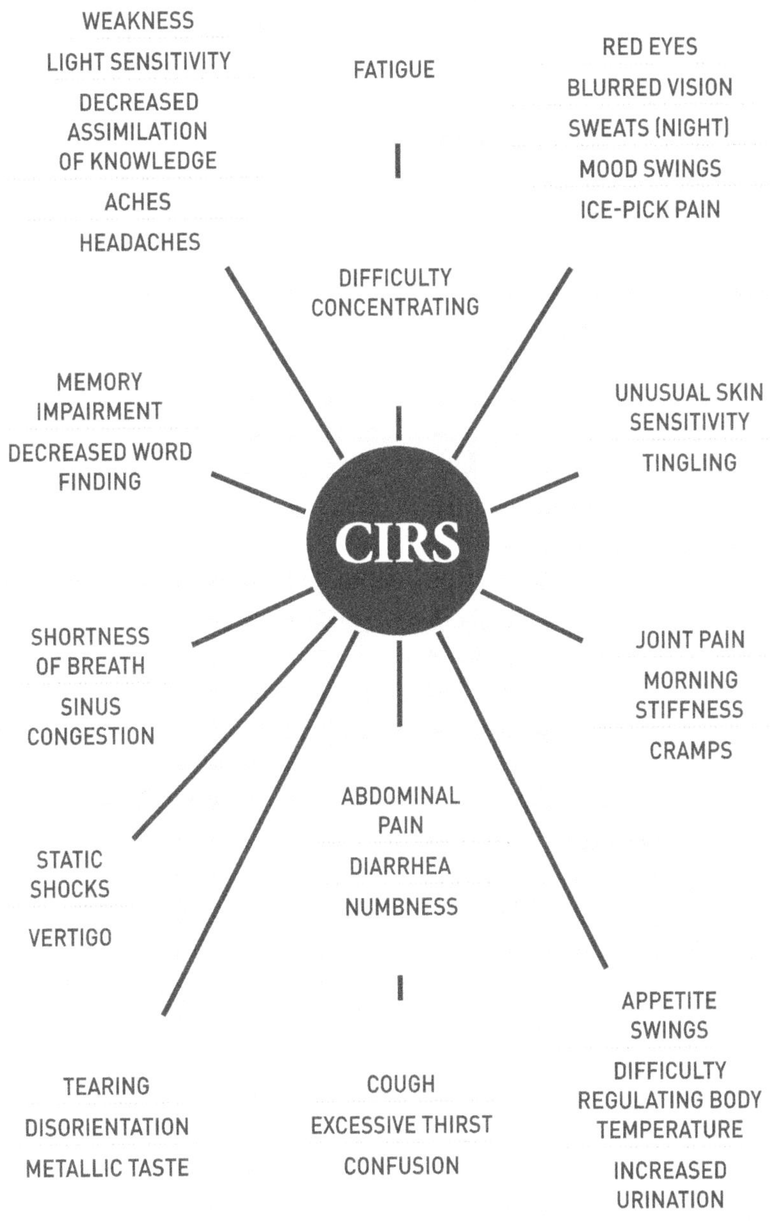

HOW DO I KNOW IF I HAVE MOULD ILLNESS?

Diagnosing biotoxin illness can be difficult, because there is no quick and easy positive/negative test that conclusively confirms biotoxin illness. Biotoxin illness is suspected if you have a chronic illness or abnormal hormone levels that haven't responded to treatment, and you have had current or past exposure to a water-damaged building. If biotoxin illness is suspected, the following methods can be used for diagnosis:

Determine if you have a history, signs, and symptoms consistent with biotoxin exposure

Have you lived in a home with a leaky roof or basement, or with visible mould? Have you been exposed to dinoflagellates or a blue green algae overgrowth? Do your symptoms get worse when you are in certain buildings? Clinical experience has shown that if you have had exposure and have symptoms from at least six of the symptom clusters above, you may have biotoxin illness, and HLA and VCS testing is warranted. (It is common to have symptoms from up to ten of the clusters.)

Confirm genetic susceptibility through an HLA-DR blood test

Those of us who carry the HLA-DR gene variation are susceptible to mould illness. It is estimated that 25% of the population has this variation, and do not make the antibodies needed to deactivate and eliminate biotoxins from mould, Lyme, and other toxic exposures, so the toxins are stored. Genetic testing can confirm whether you are in this population of people.

Take a Visual Contrast Sensitivity (VCS) Test

VCS tests measure your ability to see details at low contrast levels. Because biotoxins affect your optic nerve and decrease your ability to detect visual contrast, VCS testing is a useful screening tool to determine if you have been adversely affected by biotoxin exposure.

The VCS test is so accurate that if positive, there is a very high chance (over 90%) that you have biotoxin illness, but it is important to understand that this is not a diagnostic tool, but a screening tool. The test is done online, is inexpensive, and it only takes 10 minutes to do the test and receive your results. The VCS test is also a great tool for tracking your progress while you recover.

Take a mycotoxin test

A mycotoxin test is a simple urine test that will let you know if there is mycotoxin accumulation in your body. It is important that even if you have a high amount of mycotoxins, your test may not be positive if due to your HLA haplotype, your body is unable to tag mycotoxins as antigens. Dr. Horowitz recommends using 2000 mg of glutathione 45 minutes before the test and sweating with an infrared sauna to ensure that there is adequate movement of biotoxins. Repeating this test during treatment can help track your progress, which should coincide with improvements in your symptoms.

Take lab tests (biomarkers)

If you have a history consistent with biotoxin exposure, a susceptible genotype, and an abnormal VCS test, you are very likely to have the neuroimmune, vascular, and endocrine abnormalities that are commonly seen in biotoxin illness. How far these abnormalities have advanced can be measured through biomarkers including:

- hormones that are low (VIP, a-MSH, testosterone, ACTH, DHEA, VEGF)
- cytokines that are high (C4A, TGF-Beta 1, MMP9, MSH, leptin)
- antibodies that are high (anti-gliadin, anticardiolipin).

HOW DO I RECOVER?

Until we moved to a mould-free home:

- I had my home tested, and had all visible mould safely removed and the whole apartment fogged by experts.
- I washed all of the porous belongings that I could (such as clothes, cushions, and bedding) with baking soda, vinegar, and tea tree oil.
- I got rid of all porous items that couldn't be washed, such as books, photos, and my sofa.
- I started an organic, autoimmune Paleo, mould detox diet.

Once in our new home:

- I bought a hygrometer and a dehumidifier.
- I installed air and water filters.

- I installed moisture-sensing ventilation bathroom fans.

- I turned off our Wi-Fi and used only wired internet.

- I limited my total toxin exposure.

Treatment options for biotoxin illness

The treatment process for biotoxin illness is the same as for SIBO and heavy metals - remove the pathogens/bacteria/toxins causing you to be unwell by:

- preparing your elimination pathways
- supporting your immune system and mitochondrial function so your body can deal with the mobilised toxins and rebuild your damaged tissues and immune system
- using binders to absorb and remove the toxins (see below for more details).

It is thought that an important and sometimes overlooked step in many mould and biotoxin illness treatment protocols is the treatment of MARCoNs (Multiple Antibiotic Resistant Coagulase Negative Staphylococci).

Often, people with biotoxin illness, chronic Lyme disease, and mould exposure can develop an overgrowth of staph deep in the mucous membranes of their nose, called MARCoNs.

This is because the excessive production of inflammatory cytokines from biotoxin exposure depletes your MSH (melanocyte stimulating hormone), creating the perfect environment for bacteria to colonize and overgrow. 80% of those with low MSH are thought to have MARCoNs. (2)

Because MSH regulates hormones secreted by the pituitary gland, when your MSH falls too low, your body will respond by raising ACTH (adrenocorticotropic hormone) and cortisol to counteract the increased stress. (3) For me this manifested in very high cortisol, and serious insomnia, which resolved when I treated the MARCoNs with nasal sprays and removed/treated the underlying causes of the inflammation. Low MSH can also result in fatigue, chronic pain, hormone imbalances, mood swings, leaky gut, problems with proper bowel elimination, and low melatonin.(4)

MARCoNs is considered a controversial diagnosis because coagulase negative Staphylococci (CoNS) is often found in healthy people, particularly on the skin. (5) However, it is thought that problems arise when certain strains of potentially pathogenic bacteria overgrow and create an imbalance in your body.

It is worth noting that MARCoNS do not necessarily cause symptoms like a runny nose, sinusitis, or facial pain. A deep nasal swab and culture can determine if you have levels of MARCoNs that requires treatment. It is important to work with a medical professional who is familiar with MARCoNs, and can help you with this infection, and its root cause

Binders

For centuries, people have used various compounds to bind toxins from food, chemicals, drugs, and other harmful substances. They are also now used to bind heavy metals, pesticides, radioactive elements, and mycotoxins. These binders help your body to reduce toxins and are a critical part of any detox protocol.

When the liver processes toxins, they are excreted through your bile and into your small intestine. If the toxins are not bound to anything, most of them will be reabsorbed in your gut. Binders can be used to bind the toxins so that they can pass through the digestive tract safely and be eliminated, not reabsorbed.

A variety of different binders are available, and they each have an affinity for binding different toxins based on their net charge and molecular bonds. You can buy them individually or use a mixture of different ones, including cholestyramine, Welchol, activated charcoal, bentonite clay, zeolite, modified citrus pectin, and BioActive Carbon.

Although all binders have some benefits, many aren't very effective. Most are only able to bind certain toxins, will only work under certain conditions, and can't move beyond your gut. As well, most binders don't provide the materials required to repair the damage caused by the toxins they're getting rid of. For these reasons, the best binders are made from BioActive Carbon, because they do what you want them to, without any drawbacks.

The binders I used, Microbe Formulas' BioActive Carbon binders, are made from humic and fulvic acids that have been extracted, purified, and formulated into a binder that can bind heavy metals, pesticides, chemicals, radioactive elements, and mycotoxins. Unlike many other binders, BioActive Carbon has long-chain carbons that work in your gut as well as medium and short chain carbons that can work systemically in your cells and tissues. It only binds and removes what your body doesn't need, so you can safely take these binders with food long-term.

Research Nutritionals also has a formula called ToxinPul, which also utilises humic/fulvic acids.

It is important to work with your practitioner to ascertain which binders are suitable for you, based on your clinical history, toxic exposures, and tolerance, and which are suitable to use along with your other treatments.

Do binders interfere with supplements and medications?

Most binders easily attach to different substances. When I used activated charcoal, Welchol, and zeolites, I took them on an empty stomach either one hour before or two hours after medications and supplements to reduce the chance they would them. As mentioned, this is not an issue with Microbe Formulas' BioActive Carbon binders.

Please note that constipation is a common side effect of using binders. To avoid this, I drank a large glass of water with each dose.

Other ways to deal with constipation:

• Take Microbe Formulas' Intestinal Mover.
• Take magnesium citrate.
• Do an epsom salt flush.

- Take Vitamin C.
- Use a squatty potty.

OTHER DETOX STRATEGIES TO CONSIDER:

Glutathione

Glutathione is a naturally occurring, intracellular, master antioxidant, and people recovering from biotoxin illness often have lower levels. If your body isn't producing enough glutathione, you cannot get rid of toxins as well as other people, and they are stored in your fats and tissues and build up. When this happens, as the need and length of time to detoxify increases, your health declines. Having healthy glutathione levels is an essential part of recovering from biotoxin illness.

I take MaxOne, which naturally increases intracellular glutathione. Because of sulphur sensitivity, I cannot tolerate liposomal glutathione. Coffee enemas are also thought to be an excellent way to detoxify your body through enhancing your body's detoxifying enzyme systems in your intestines and liver. It is believed that they also open your bile duct system, which will flush stagnant bile from your liver and gallbladder. (6).

Infrared sauna

Studies have found that increased sweating can help you excrete toxins. Saunas are an excellent way to do this, and infrared saunas can help you sweat at a much faster rate than traditional saunas, as the infrared heat penetrates your body more deeply. It is important to use one that has low EMFs and is made from non-toxic materials.

Antifungals

When people start to get sick from mould, their good bacteria has difficulty competing with the mycotoxins, and so they often develop candida. Anti-fungals that will help kill candida and help you regain better-balanced bacteria include:

- Nystatin
- garlic
- oregano oil
- pau d'arco
- olive leaf extract
- caprylic acid
- barberry
- grapefruit seed extract.

Rotating them to avoid the candida becoming resistant as it mutates will give you the best results. There are also many pharmaceuticals that are useful in resistant patients, so if this is you, please consult your medical professional.

HOW DO I KNOW IF THERE IS MOULD IN MY HOME?

It is important to be aware of the warning signs that you may be sharing your home with more than just your family. Mould is not always visible; it can live within your walls, ceiling, or beneath wallpaper, tiles, or linoleum, so you may not even be aware that there is a problem.

In addition to the visible appearance of mould in places such as your bathroom, kitchen, basement or cellar, corners and dark areas, other signs that there may be a mould issue are:

* musty or dank smell in your home
* water damage from a leak or flood
* you or other members of your household have experienced symptoms of mould-related illness.

Mould can be dangerous to your health and become a serious issue very quickly if left untreated, so you need to be aggressive in locating the source. Surface mould can be cleaned with many common natural cleaners, but internal mould or serious water damage should always be handled by an experienced company, or it will just keep coming back and getting worse.

If you suffer from allergies or someone in your home is showing symptoms of mould illness or allergy, it might be wise to find a temporary place to stay until the problem is dealt with, so that you aren't exposed to disrupted mould spores. Many people choose to stay elsewhere while the mould is remediated in their homes.

Hire a certified mould inspector or building biologist

It is possible to remove mould from your home by yourself, but if you are suffering from mould illness, it is not recommended. The process of getting rid of mould disturbs the spores, and sends them floating around, which can worsen any health problems you have.

If you see mould in one part of your home, there is a good chance it is in other areas that are not readily visible. For instance, it can grow inside walls and heating and ventilation ducts, and is difficult to remove from those areas. Not removing the mould completely will cause your health issues to continue, so it is best to get the job done correctly the first time by someone who has experience in this area.

The recommended way to determine if there is a mould problem in your home is to hire a certified mould inspector or building biologist trained in mould testing. Don't choose a mould inspector based on price alone. Many mould inspectors do not use comprehensive, accurate testing methods, and will only do a visual inspection and take some air samples. Both methods can be useful but on their own, they are not enough.

Air sampling does not pick up some mould species, and air sampling devices only collect a small sample directly around the device. This is important because some mould spores do not remain airborne for long and they may not be sampling near the source of the issue. A better method of screening for mould is the ERMI test, which can identify mould in dust that has settled around your home.

For these reasons, it is best if the person you have chosen has a background in biological sciences and building sciences, and that they are properly trained and experienced in investigating and sampling mould and in how to interpret the lab results. They can use infrared cameras to find hidden moisture, produce a moisture map for you, and can provide you with a comprehensive inspection report documenting their visual findings, environmental monitoring results, interpretation of lab results, and their conclusions and recommendations on how to control/remediate the mould problem.

If you own your home, you will have to cover the costs of inspection and clean-up. However, if you rent, your property owner should take care of the problem for you, as mould is now a recognised health hazard.

HOW DO I SAFELY KILL MOULD MYSELF?

If assessment shows that the only mould in your home is on hard surfaces like bathtubs or the grout on your kitchen tiles, you can remove it effectively with any of the following natural household cleaners. They don't contain harsh chemicals, produce dangerous fumes, or leave behind toxic residue, so they are safe for your family, pets, and the environment. You can apply them directly to the mould and allow them to soak before wiping off the mould.

Vinegar

Vinegar is a powerful antifungal and antibacterial, and is an inexpensive way to kill many mould species. It is readily available, non-toxic, and can be sprayed on most surfaces. Important note: Never mix vinegar with bleach. Doing so can produce chlorine gas.

Baking Soda

Baking soda is another well-known, inexpensive household cleaner
that you can also use to kill mould. Baking soda also deodorizes,
which helps to get rid of any musty smells, and it absorbs moisture,
which helps keep mould away. Vinegar and baking soda are often
used together when cleaning up a mould problem, as vinegar kills
different species of mould than baking soda.

Hydrogen Peroxide

Hydrogen peroxide is an anti-fungal, anti-viral, and anti-bacterial,
and kills mould effectively on many materials. It is a good alternative
to chlorine bleach because it doesn't produce toxic fumes, leave
toxic residue behind, or damage the environment. It is inexpensive
and is a bleaching agent, so it can help fade the stains that mould
leaves behind. It is a good idea to spot test it on any material you are
cleaning to make sure it will not fade the colour.

Borax

Although borax is toxic if you swallow it, it does not emit chemicals
or dangerous fumes like some other mould killers. This white
mineral powder has a low toxicity and is used as a deodorizer,
insecticide, herbicide, and fungicide and can be mixed with water
in a solution to kill and remove mould. You can buy borax at the
supermarket in the laundry section.

Essential oils

Studies show that many essential oils are anti-fungal and will kill mould. Some of the best options are tea tree oil, oregano, thyme, cinnamon, and clove oils. A great way to hit the mould directly is to use a spray bottle and a mixture of essential oil and either vinegar or isopropyl alcohol and water.

Colloidal Silver

Colloidal silver is a powerful and effective anti-fungal, and can be used undiluted to spray on an affected area.

WHY SHOULDN'T I USE BLEACH OR AMMONIA?

Bleach

Although sodium hypochlorite, the active ingredient in bleach, is the main ingredient in many mould removal products, there are many reasons to use safer alternatives.

- Bleach is a harsh and corrosive chemical that gives off fumes, and produces toxic gas when combined with ammonia.
- Bleach cannot completely kill mould that is growing in porous materials such as drywall or wood.
- The chlorine in bleach stays on the surface of a material, while absorbing the water component, further feeding the mould. Although the mould on the surface is killed, the roots are left intact, and the mould can quickly return.

For these reasons try to avoid using bleach, but if you do, only use it on non-porous surfaces.

Ammonia

Like bleach, ammonia will kill mould on non-porous surfaces, but it is also a harsh, toxic chemical. Make sure you never mix ammonia with bleach, because the gas they create when combined is toxic.

How to clean

- Protect yourself by wearing a respirator, goggles, and gloves.
- Vacuum the affected area with a HEPA vacuum to remove the mould spores.
- Wipe the affected area using microfibre cloths and your chosen cleaner.
- Throw away or disinfect the cloths immediately after use to prevent the spread of active mould spores.

A three-bucket system works well:

1. Rinse your soiled/contaminated cloth in a bucket of water to get rid of most of the particles and mould.

2. More thoroughly rinse your cloth in a second bucket with a mix of 80% vinegar/20% water.

3. Dip your 'cleaned' cloth into a third bucket of fresh 80% vinegar/20% water for more cleaning.

HOW DO I PREVENT MOULD?

Once your home has been remediated, or if you have moved into a new mould-free home, there are many things you can do to ensure your living space remains safe and mould-free.

While you may feel overwhelmed when reading this list for the first time, just try addressing the recommendations one at a time.

Balance the humidity with a hygrometer and dehumidifier

Mould grows in relative humidity of 60% and over, so a dehumidifier can be a useful tool in keeping the humidity in your home at low levels, especially in damp areas such as the basement and bathroom.

I use a hygrometer to measure the humidity in my home. There are many inexpensive ones available online. I prefer the humidity in my home to be around 50%, and when it rises much more than that, I run my dehumidifier until it drops to desired levels.

In choosing a dehumidifier, it is important to choose the right model for your home, climate, and intended use. I found it helpful to call a company that produces dehumidifiers to talk through all the things I needed to consider.

Purify your water

Your tap water can contain things like mould, chlorine, pesticides, heavy metals, and fluoride. These toxins can affect your wellbeing, as your body has to work hard to get rid of them. There are many types of water purifiers that you can buy to remove these things from the water you drink, cook with, or wash with. You can purchase whole-house, under-sink, shower, or counter-top systems.

Because I live in a rented home, I use a counter-top Travel Berkey. When filled, it easily provides enough filtered water for two of us for daily drinking and cooking. I also use a Sonaki VitaPure inline shower filter, which I was able to easily exchange for the shower head that was provided and that I can also take when we leave.

'Scrub' your air

Air purifiers can clean and sanitize the air and surfaces in your home, and make it healthier by safely removing mould spores, allergens, and bacteria. There are many other indoor air contaminants worth being concerned about as well, so one of the best things you can invest in is a high-quality air filter for your home. Recommended brands include Air Oasis, IQ Air and Austin Air Purifiers.

Ventilate your bathroom

Mould loves moisture, so bathrooms are vulnerable to mould growth. A bathroom ventilation fan is a great tool to prevent this, especially in modern apartments that do not have a bathroom window. First, ensure that the fan is ducted to the exterior of your home. Fans can be controlled by the same switch that operates your bathroom lights, but it is preferable to install a fan that is controlled by a humidistat.

The humidistat will measure the humidity level in your bathroom and turn the fan on when a pre-set humidity level is detected. It will then turn the fan off automatically when the humidity falls below that pre-set level.

Use an effective, all-purpose cleaning spray

I use a general, non-toxic cleaning spray everywhere in my home, including on the tiles, glass, and cupboards in the kitchen and bathroom, as well as on walls and furniture. This all-purpose cleaning spray also kills mould. I make it myself from the following inexpensive, readily available ingredients, and keep it in a spray bottle:

- 2 cups distilled white vinegar
- 2 teaspoons tea tree essential oil.

Kill unwanted pathogens in your laundry

I add 1/2 cup baking soda, 1/2 teaspoon tea tree oil, and 1-2 cups of vinegar to every load of washing I do. As well as removing residue, stains, mould and bacteria, vinegar works as a clothes softener. Another product you can use to remove mould is borax. Use half a cup of borax in hot water (to make sure it dissolves) when washing your clothes.

Diffuse mould-killing essential oils

Diffusing essential oils is an effective way to prevent mould in your home. I use a nebulising diffuser because it does not require water to operate, so it does not add any moisture to the air. The following oils are known to be effective:

- cinnamon
- thyme
- clove
- tea tree oil
- DoTerra On-Guard (this is my favourite).

Other general tips to avoid mould growth:

- Immediately clean and dry any spills.
- Vacuum your home regularly, especially if you have carpet.
- Ensure air flows and circulates regularly through your home.
- Keep the clothes in your closet dry and clean, and avoid overcrowding.
- Place your furniture slightly away from walls to allow for better air flow.
- Check the soil of your houseplants.

MONTHLY MAINTENANCE SCHEDULE

For those of us with biotoxin illness, preventing mould exposure is essential. Every month, I check all the areas in my home where mould commonly grows.

While doing all of these things may seem daunting, especially when you have such little energy to get through everything else, keeping on top of them will help you recover quicker. You don't have to do them all on the same day. You will find that you get in the swing of whatever routine you develop, and once you have done them each a couple of times, they will become easier. You will feel more relaxed just knowing your environment is 'safe'. I always protect myself by wearing a respirator, goggles, and gloves when doing any of the maintenance cleaning.

Do visual inspections of the places mould likes to grow

It is important to periodically check all the places that mould might like to grow, especially in the winter when heating causes condensation, and in the summer when the humidity is high. I do a visual check monthly of door and window frames, behind bulkheads, on the tops and backs of blinds, on all grout and tiles, and anywhere water can pool, such as behind the bathroom sink and the kitchen mixer tap.

Keep the drains clean

When water, food, hair, or other things sit in your drains, mould can grow. To keep my drains clean and mould-free, I pour ½ cup baking soda down the bathroom and kitchen drains and let it sit overnight. This starts to kill the mould and dry up the slime. The next day, I pour 2 cups of white vinegar or hydrogen peroxide down the same drains and watch it foam. This kills the mould and loosens the mould colony's hold on the pipes. Then I pour 5-6 cups of very hot water down the drains to wash away the dead mould, baking soda, and vinegar or hydrogen peroxide. Note - Do not use boiling water because it can damage your pipes and connections, especially if they are made of PVC.

Check all large home appliances

Because large home appliances such as washing machines, dishwashers, and refrigerators all have water and many dark nooks and crannies where mould could thrive, it is important to check them regularly, to prevent mould growth, or catch it early.

Washing machine

As well as inside the folds of the door seal of front loaders or in the space between the tubs in top loaders, there are other places in washing machines that mould can flourish, such as in the pipes and other nooks and crannies.

I bought an Asko washer, and although expensive, Askos do not have rubber door seals. The inner and outer drums are both made of stainless steel, so it does not have the mould build-up that usually occurs with front loaders.

I still leave the detergent drawer and door wide open after every wash, clean out the pin trap and dispenser drawer, and run the machine through a drum wash with 1-2 cups of baking soda and 1-2 cups of white vinegar monthly.

Dishwasher

You'd think that with the amount of water that runs through dishwashers, mould might be a common issue in the corrugated water pipes. However, the food trap located in the floor of the machine needs to be regularly taken apart and cleaned, because food and grease can collect there and start to rot. Besides keeping the food trap clean, I slide the dishwasher out fully to make sure there are no leaks behind or beneath it. I also run a cycle on the hottest setting monthly, with 1-2 cups of baking soda and 1-2 cups of vinegar.

You can buy a dishwasher pan so that if there is a leak, water condensation, or hose failure, the water will not soak into the floor, back wall, and cabinets. For added protection, you can also put an electric leak detector in the pan.

Refrigerator

Mould can grow behind a refrigerator, as well as inside it. Moisture, plus a lack of ventilation, provides ideal conditions for mould growth inside, especially in the door seals. Warmth generated by the compressor, typical kitchen humidity, and the moisture created by the evaporative coils create ideal conditions for mould to grow behind your refrigerator. It is important to inspect for and clean any that you find.

If you have an ice or water dispenser, you need to clean all the tubes with vinegar and water. Remove those you can and use a cotton swab for hard-to-reach places such as the water dispenser faucet. If your refrigerator has an air filter, change it every three to six months. I pull the refrigerator out and clean the drip pan monthly, and keep the refrigerator pulled out slightly from the wall to improve air circulation.

Air conditioner

Mould can grow almost anywhere, and if it gets inside your heating or air-conditioning system, it will spread throughout the house. I have a split heating/cooling system, so I regularly take off the front cover, remove the filters, soak them with vinegar and baking soda, vacuum the inside of the unit, then drain and let the filters dry, and reinstall them.

Keep known problem areas mould-free

We live in a modern apartment with a bathroom that has no window and poor air circulation. Even though I run a dehumidifier for two hours every morning after I shower, and our bathroom has a ventilation fan, I still find that after a number of weeks, scum starts to form on the shower floor and in the corners of the shower. I know that if I left this for long enough, mould would grow. I find that using a homemade cleaning paste is extremely effective in keeping our bathroom mould-free.

I make this paste from baking soda mixed with just enough vinegar to make it spreadable. I smear this on tiles in the shower recess, and on the tile floor. I let it sit for at least an hour, then use a scrubbing brush to vigorously scour the tiles and grout.

Watch for musty smells in your car

Because cars are sealed up, get warm inside, and lack ventilation, given the right conditions, mould can easily start to grow in your car. Contributing factors include spilled liquids, forgotten food, living in a humid climate, condensation, spores coming in through the air conditioner, the car being stored in a damp garage, rain, or flood damage. Musty smells are a clue that something is growing in your car that shouldn't be there.

To clean your car, put on your respirator, and do the following:

- If possible, move your car into direct sunlight.
- Open all the doors and windows and air it out for at least 30 minutes.
- Remove everything that you can, and inspect the car interior carefully for any visible mould, and vacuum with a HEPA vacuum.
- Use your all-purpose cleaning spray on all surfaces, using a toothbrush to get into hard-to-reach places.

To clean inside your car's climate control system:

- Close the doors and windows, turn the fan to high, and make sure that you set it to fresh, so it is not recirculating the internal air.
- Standing outside your car, hold a tissue over the outside vent near your windscreen wiper.
- Where you see air being pulled in, spray a generous amount of your

general mould cleaning spray to allow it to be pulled into the vent system and into your car.

- Open the car doors, and leave the fan running for ten minutes.
- Spray the inside of all your air vents with cleaning spray, close the doors and windows and run the AC on circulation for five minutes.

Preventative measures:

- Be diligent about cleaning up any moisture.
- Open the windows and air out your car often.
- Use a car air purifier or a diffuser with a mould-killing essential oil when you drive.
- Keep moisture absorbers in your car.
- Keep your car rubbish free, and clean the interior regularly.
- Mist with your general mould spray and 'fog' your car monthly.

THE CONNECTION BETWEEN MOULD ILLNESS AND LYME DISEASE

Mould illness and Lyme disease are both biotoxin illnesses. Many patients will have CIRS related to water damaged buildings as well as CIRS related to Lyme, as the HLA genes for both overlap significantly.

Getting sick with Lyme disease can also trigger mould illness, as borrelia bacteria produce biotoxins that can induce CIRS, making the home you previously tolerated too toxic for you.

HELPFUL REFERENCES AND RESOURCES

1. Dr. Horowitz's Sixteen-Point Differential Diagnosis MSIDS Map can be found in his book, Horowitz, Richard I M.D. 2017. *How Can I Get Better? An Action Plan for Treating Resistant Lyme and Chronic Disease*, St. Martin's Griffin, New York, New York, p 50-65

2. *Inquiry into Biotoxin-related Illnesses in Australia, Submission 129.* Australian Chronic Infectious & Inflammatory Disease Society, 2018.

3. Allen MJ, Sharma S. *Physiology, Adrenocorticotropic Hormone (ACTH)* [Updated 2021 Aug 17]. In: StatPearls [Internet]. Treasure Island (FL): StatPearls Publishing; 2021 Jan.

4. Natasha Thomas, M.D. *Understanding Chronic Inflammatory Response Syndrome (CIRS).*2016.

5. Becker K, Heilmann C, Peters G. *Coagulase-negative staphylococci.* Clin Microbiol Rev. 2014;27(4):870-926. doi:10.1128/CMR.00109-13.

6. Gerson Institute 1993-1999, *Gerson Therapy Handbook*, Revised Fifth Edition, Gerson Institute.

Neil Nathan, MD - https://neilnathanmd.com

Neil Nathan, M.D. has been working to raise awareness that mould toxicity is a major contributing factor for patients with chronic illness.

Dr Nathan lectures internationally on this subject, which led to the publication of his book, *Mold and Mycotoxins: Current Evaluation and Treatment*, 2016. His most recent book *Toxic: Heal Your Body from Mold Toxicity, Lyme Disease, Multiple Chemical Sensitivities, and Chronic Environmental Illness* is intended help people understand the causes of their illness and how to heal from them.

www.survivingmold.com

This resource is a partnership between Dr. Shoemaker and a family who has recovered from mould illness. Their goal is to provide help, information, and hope for those who are suffering.

www.microbeformulas.com

The Microbe Formulas website is my all-time favourite health resource for information on heavy metal toxicity, mould illness, parasites, Lyme disease and co-infections. On their site, Dr. Todd Watts and Dr. Jay Davidson of Microbe Formulas provide numerous videos and articles. You can search the Learn section by topic and find informative and enlightening resource materials as well as effective treatment and maintenance protocol advice. The support team at Microbe Formulas are fantastic. I called them many times to ask numerous questions about their products and treatment protocols, and I can't recommend them highly enough.

‘YOU CANNOT PREVENT
THE BIRDS OF
SORROW FROM FLYING
OVER YOUR HEAD, BUT
YOU CAN PREVENT
THEM FROM BUILDING
NESTS IN YOUR HAIR.’

CHINESE PROVERB

CHAPTER SIX

PARASITES
A COMMONLY OVERLOOKED ISSUE

I USED TO THINK THAT PARASITES WERE ONLY FOUND IN DEVELOPING COUNTRIES OR IN UNHYGIENIC CONDITIONS, BUT IT TURNS OUT THAT THEY ARE VERY COMMON, ANYONE CAN HAVE THEM, AND THEY ARE NOT EASILY DIAGNOSED BECAUSE OF THE WIDE RANGE OF SYMPTOMS YOU MAY HAVE, AND BECAUSE OF DIFFICULTIES IN TESTING. IF YOU THINK THAT IT IS UNLIKELY THAT PARASITES ARE PART OF YOUR HEALTH ISSUES, THINK AGAIN.

I learned that parasites enter our bodies easily through our water, food, environment, and pets, and they play a part in almost every chronic illness. Just thinking about this made me cringe. It was creepy to think about these critters living it up inside me, but I finally understood how widespread parasites are, and why it was so important to clear them.

For years, I'd had extreme digestive symptoms. When they first appeared, I couldn't sit down for more than an hour or two through the entire day, or the fermentation would quickly build up in my intestines, causing pain. I belched around the clock. It was excruciatingly embarrassing, especially at work. My colleagues knew

I had a 'medical condition' and would kindly pretend they couldn't hear me belching as I worked. I scheduled multiple walks around the block throughout the day so I could sit down for one-hour meetings. At night, I had to walk for at least an hour and belch constantly, to settle things enough to get to sleep. It was exhausting.

Almost all foods made it worse, especially fats. The only foods I tolerated well were chicken, zucchini, and carrots. Those three foods became every meal for me, with the only variation being what shape I cut the vegetables into. For special occasions, I cut them into stars.

Doctors would just look at me quizzically when I explained the severity of the symptoms. More than one doctor suggested that my excessive belching was from swallowing too much air when I ate, or that anxiety was causing me to swallow more often. Over the years, I was tested and treated for h pylori, candida, SIBO, and gut dysbiosis.

With each diagnosis came the feeling of hope that this was the answer to my digestive issues, but five years and many rounds of antimicrobial and antibacterial treatments later, the symptoms had reduced to about 30%, but were still relentless. My instincts told me that aside from the unhealthy terrain of my gut, there was still something my doctors hadn't found. What I have learned since then is that more than half of us will pick up parasites at some point, especially those of us with immune dysfunction due to Lyme disease, other pathogens, or toxins.

As parasite expert Dr. Todd Watts says, 'If you have a pulse, you have parasites'. He believes that to fully recover from chronic illness, you need to start by clearing your parasites. This is because your immune system cannot clear viruses and bacteria, while it is being affected by parasites.

Another thing I came to understand is that parasites can cause many symptoms, of which only a few are digestive. I was surprised to learn that as well as being in our guts, parasites can also be in our circulatory and lymphatic systems, brain, spinal cord, central nervous system, lungs, eyes, liver, nasal cavity and sinuses, and ears. This is because their long reproduction cycles and migration tendencies take them all over our bodies, where they take hold and wreak havoc.

The symptoms are varied and extensive and like many of those you experience in Lyme disease. They can vary from minor to extreme, including fatigue, brain fog, muscle and joint pain, insomnia, skin, and digestive issues. The process of treating parasites can take from six months to three years, depending on the severity of your infection and how long you have had it. About 70% of parasites are microscopic, but some, like huge tapeworms, can grow to over 30 meters in length.

Take heart in knowing that you can clear parasites from your body, and in doing so, will resolve many different symptoms and health issues. The critical thing to remember is the importance of continuing to 'take out the trash', and that even when you feel the issue is resolved, you introduce a maintenance protocol.

I used the Microbe Formulas treatment protocol to treat my parasite infection. From the very first dose of anti-parasitic herbs, I saw visible evidence of parasites, after years of being told my stool tests were normal. I spent many months focussed on getting rid of them, and in doing so, I finally made huge leaps in my overall recovery

.

THE PRACTICAL STUFF

HOW DO I KNOW IF I HAVE PARASITES?

Testing for parasites is tricky, and they frequently go undetected. Parasites may not come out in all your bowel movements, and if your stool isn't viewed immediately after you collect your sample, the lab may not see anything. This is because parasites release enzymes that start to dissolve their body once they die, and by the time your sample reaches the lab, the evidence is gone. In addition, there are thousands of different types of parasites, but tests only check for a few common ones, so getting tested can be a waste of time.

HOW DO I TREAT PARASITES?

A good place to start with parasite treatment is with changes to your diet, by removing the things parasites thrive on, such as grains, sugars, and processed foods. Introducing things such as vitamin C, garlic, cinnamon, apple cider vinegar, coconut oil, and pumpkin seeds can help boost your ability to fight back. Following that, there are several proven herbal and holistic treatments that you can use to treat parasites.

However, it is important to note that some people have food sensitivities and cannot tolerate things like garlic or coconut. It is important to be checked for both IgE and IgG food allergies, leaky gut, and histamine sensitivity with mast cell activation.

Dr. Hulda Clark was one of the first people to make a connection between chronic illness and parasites. She recommends a combination of black walnut hulls, wormwood, and clove to rid the body of many different infections without negative side effects. Another powerful treatment for parasites is mimosa pudica, which paralyses parasites so you can then eliminate them in your bowel movements.

Microbe Formulas have developed a very high quality, organic mimosa pudica seed product as well as two other products, Formula 1 and 2, that help evict any unwanted guests. I have used all three products to effectively combat both intestinal and systemic parasites, as part of doing the overall Microbe Formulas treatment protocol. It is important to note that while this may be helpful, it may not be enough for some common parasites found in Lyme patients, such as Babesia, and you may require additional treatment.

When you start treatment, you need to be aware that as you kill the parasites, you will also release the pathogens and toxins they have been shielding. To avoid severe die-off reactions, it is important that you follow a comprehensive protocol, as with treating heavy metal toxicity, SIBO, and biotoxin illness. This includes:

- preparing your elimination pathways
- supporting your immune system and mitochondrial function so your body can deal with the mobilised toxins and rebuild your damaged tissues and immune system
- using fulvic acid and carbon-based binders to absorb and remove the toxins.

HELPFUL RESOURCE

www.microbeformulas.com

The Microbe Formulas website is my all-time favourite health resource for information on heavy metal toxicity, mould illness, parasites, Lyme disease and co-infections. On their site, Dr. Todd Watts and Dr. Jay Davidson of Microbe Formulas provide numerous videos and articles. You can search the Learn section by topic and find informative and enlightening resource materials as well as effective treatment and maintenance protocol advice. The support team at Microbe Formulas are fantastic. I called them many times to ask numerous questions about their products and treatment protocols, and I can't recommend them highly enough.

'SO FAR YOU HAVE
SURVIVED 100% OF
YOUR WORST DAYS.
YOU ARE DOING GREAT.'

UNKNOWN

CHAPTER SEVEN

LYME DISEASE
AND CO-INFECTIONS

THE WORDS OF ANOTHER PSYCHIC NEARLY 25 YEARS LATER LED TO THE DIAGNOSIS THAT CHANGED EVERYTHING. SHE SAID, 'YOU HAVE LYME. YOU GOT IT WHEN YOU WERE SIX YEARS OLD. YOU LIVED SOMEWHERE FLAT, WITH SHALLOW BEACHES AND FOREST. YOU NEED TO GET TESTED.'

She perfectly described the island where I lived when I was six. I reminisced about the amount of time I spent as a child outdoors at the beach and in the forest on our farm. Although my mother can remember removing a tick from one of my brothers, she doesn't recall doing the same for me. I have no doubt that I was bitten by many things during those years though.

Until now, my other diagnoses seemed like legitimate reasons for most of the symptoms I had been struggling with. Because testing for Lyme disease is complicated and expensive, and I thought Lyme was rare, I had never considered being tested for it before.

However, the reality was that even after years of heavy metal chelation, and 18-months of binding mould toxins, I didn't really feel much better yet. I was still underweight, exhausted but unable to sleep well, experiencing brain fog, relentless digestive distress, muscle and joint pain, and fighting a 'virus' that brought night sweats, fever, sore throat and swollen glands on a weekly cycle. I felt terrible all the time, and despite living so close to the beach, found it too difficult to even drag myself there many days, despite how good it felt to get into the ocean.

For years, my instincts had been that there was still something undiagnosed. Not having had much luck with getting answers through the medical professionals I was consulting with, I decided to see a psychic. When she told me that I had Lyme disease, her words went struck me deeply and I finally decided to seek out a doctor proficient in testing for and treating Lyme. I asked my GP who to see to be tested and diagnosed for Lyme, and he said that the man I wanted to see was Dr. Geoff Kemp, an expert in the diagnosis and treatment of Lyme, with over 50 years' experience as a doctor.

My first appointment with the Dr. Kemp, went on for hours. He very patiently collected my health history and took the time to discuss my symptoms in detail. His knowledge about Lyme is immense and he matched all my symptoms either to Lyme or one of its co-infections. He explained how Lyme could also be the underlying reason for the development and severity of the other illnesses I'd had through my life, such as glandular fever (mononucleosis) and cold sores, because of its effect on my immune system. As we talked, my whole body relaxed. Finally, I was in the treatment rooms of someone who not only recognised exactly what was causing all my symptoms, but also for whom I was not an unusual patient. I cried with relief on the way home.

My health improved more in the first four months of the Microbe Formulas treatment protocol than in the many years before. As with other pathogens, infections, and toxins, resolving Lyme disease depends on using an effective approach. This included supporting my detox pathways and mitochondrial energy, killing off parasites before killing the Lyme bacteria, and mopping up the toxins produced along the way.

However, it is important to note that an essential aspect of fully recovering people's health is addressing biofilms and persister forms of Borrelia burgdorferi, as they drive a lot of the inflammation in the body. Persister forms do not respond to standard antibiotics, and using herbal protocols alone is almost never enough, so it is important to incorporate specific persister treatments into your regimen. (1)

THE PRACTICAL STUFF

WHAT IS LYME DISEASE?

Lyme disease is a multi-system infectious disease caused by *Borrelia burgdorferi* bacteria. Once considered rare, Lyme is exploding around the world.

When you are bitten by an infected tick, it transmits *Borrelia burgdorferi* during the feeding process. If your immune system responds immediately, acute symptoms will occur. However, Borrelia's complex characteristics often allow it to evade detection by your immune system and persist in your body. If your immune system does not quickly detect the bacteria, or if treatment during the acute phase does not work, you may have chronic symptoms. If it goes undiagnosed, you can live in a cycle of managing symptoms without ever getting well.

Reports of Lyme disease began to emerge in the 1960s and 1970s in the United States. In 1975, when numerous people in Lyme and Old Lyme, Connecticut came down with fatigue, arthritis and neurological symptoms, the medical community started to pay attention. Research led to the discovery that these people had all had tick bites before their symptoms began. In 1981, Willy Burgdorfer, a Swiss-American scientist, discovered that the cause of Lyme disease was a spirochete, which he named *Borrelia burgdorferi*.

Lyme disease facts:

- Global warming has meant that tick reproductive rates are higher, they are emerging earlier each year, and that they are spreading to places they haven't been in the past, meaning an increase in infections.

- A tick bite will not always produce a bullseye rash, and some people may not notice the rash. It is thought that around 50% of people will get a rash, but only half of them look like bullseye rashes. The numbers are as low as 10% up to 80% in the scientific literature.

- The standard antibody blood test for Lyme disease has an estimated accuracy of less than 50%, especially if you are tested soon after being bitten.

- Over 150 symptoms are associated with Lyme disease, which is why it is often called 'the great imitator'. Patients are often misdiagnosed, because it produces symptoms that mimic other conditions such as arthritis, fibromyalgia, chronic fatigue syndrome, MS, and lupus.

- Ticks can also pass on bacterial, parasitic, and viral infections at the same time as Lyme disease. If you have Lyme, there's a strong chance you also have co-infections that need to be treated.

- There are over 300 strains of Borrelia around the world, which makes testing and diagnosis challenging.

- Lyme disease has four forms, spirochetes, cyst/round body, intracellular, and biofilm/persister forms, and they ALL must be treated.

- The sooner Lyme disease is detected, the easier it generally is to treat. Soon after infection you may have flu-like symptoms.

- Chronic Lyme disease (also called late Lyme) may appear over time especially if your Lyme disease was not fully eliminated with earlier treatment.

WHY IS LYME CONTROVERSIAL?

Since it was discovered, Lyme disease has been plagued by controversy. Part of the issue lies with there being two conflicting sets of guidelines for the diagnosis and treatment of Lyme. One set was developed by The Infectious Diseases Society of America (IDSA), and another by the International Lyme and Associated Diseases Society (ILADS).

Many healthcare professionals in the mainstream medical community still believe that Lyme disease is rare, easy to diagnose, and can be easily treated with a short round of antibiotics, as reflected by the IDSA guidelines.

However, there is a significant amount of evidence that Lyme disease is an extremely common yet complex condition that can become chronic, that existing testing is unreliable, and treatment needs to be tailored to the patient's response. The ILADS guidelines reflect this, and recommend the need for clinical diagnosis, recognise that some patients need higher doses and longer treatment, and that there is a chronic form of the disease.

Because of these opposing guidelines, healthcare professionals find it confusing to know the best way to test for and treat Lyme disease, and fear investigations and censure if they treat outside the IDSA guidelines. Therefore, the screening and protocol used by many of them continues to deprive people of the diagnosis and treatment they need to get better. (3)

WHAT ARE THE SYMPTOMS OF LYME DISEASE?

Two of the most well-recognised indications that you might have contracted Lyme disease are a recent tick bite or a 'bull's-eye' rash. However few people notice or remember a tick bite, and in many cases, there is no rash.

The other symptoms you may have can be vague, inconsistent, diverse, and numerous. This is because of the way that Borrelia burgdorferi causes inflammation, downregulates immunity, and provokes autoimmunity. Also, because everyone has a range of different co-infections with their Lyme disease, it does not follow a predictable course. However, there are classical symptoms that are associated with Lyme disease. A hallmark of active Lyme disease is migratory joint, muscle pain, or nerve pain (tingling, numbness, burning, or stabbing sensations). Usually, women will feel worse around their menstrual cycle, and courses of antibiotics will usually make the symptoms better or worse, implying a Herxheimer reaction.

Other common symptoms of Lyme disease include:

- chronic fatigue
- autoimmune symptoms

- brain fog and cognitive issues

- skin conditions

- heart issues

- neurological disorders

- digestive issues and abdominal pain

- hair loss

- headaches, dizziness, fever

- night sweats and sleep disturbances

- rashes, tremors

- sensitivity to light and vision changes

- jaw pain, sore throat, swollen glands

- unexplained weight loss or gain

- back stiffness, pelvic pain

- bladder inflammation or irritable bladder syndrome

- eyelid/facial twitching, or swelling around your eyes.

Please note that there can be many reasons for similar symptoms. Dr. Richard Horowitz, M.D. has put together a Sixteen-Point Differential Diagnosis Map (4) which includes some of the most common differential diagnoses and medical conditions responsible for the associated symptoms. If you have unsuccessfully tried many different interventions to determine the cause of your symptoms, it can help you and your medical professionals know how to approach testing and treatment, as often there will be multiple things that need treatment.

Dr. Richard Horowitz, MD is one of the most sought out Lyme Disease doctors in the world. He is one of the founding members of ILADS (the International Lyme & Associated Diseases Society), the leader on Lyme Disease research and education.

HOW DO I KNOW I HAVE IT?

Dr. Richard Horowitz has also put together the Lyme-MSIDS Questionnaire. This validated screening tool can help you determine the probability of having Lyme and its associated co-infections. (5)

A score over 63 on the Questionnaire means that you have a high probability of having Lyme disease. You can back this up with a clinical/lab diagnosis by an experienced medical professional who is familiar with diagnosing and treating Lyme disease, and can correctly interpret your results.

Co-infections

Over 95% of people with Lyme disease have other infections. This is because vectors like ticks, mosquitos, and fleas carry bacteria, viruses, and parasites and can transmit them at the same time in a single bite, or you can acquire them from multiple bites. Diseases acquired together like this are called co-infections. People who suffer from co-infections generally are more unwell, have more symptoms, and have a more difficult recovery.

Since Lyme disease was first identified in 1981, researchers have found more than a dozen new tick-borne pathogens, and more are still being discovered. Common co-infections are Babesia, Bartonella, relapsing fever borrelia (like *Borrelia miyamotoi*), Anaplasma, tularaemia rickettsia, Ehrlichia, Mycoplasma, Epstein Barr (EBV), and human herpes virus-6 (HHV-6).

It is important that your doctor considers co-infections when diagnosing and developing your treatment plan for Lyme disease.

WHY IS LYME DISEASE HARD TO TREAT?

Lyme disease is notoriously difficult to treat because of the bacteria's ability to camouflage itself to evade your immune system, adapt to treatments, change its shape into antibiotic-resistant cysts, and exist as 'persister' forms in biofilms. Borrelia impairs your immune system, allowing the bacteria to persist in your body and make you vulnerable to opportunistic infections.

Therefore, treatment of Lyme disease needs to be holistic, and as with other toxins and pathogens, include:

• preparing and supporting your elimination/detox pathways

• supporting your immune system and mitochondrial function so your body can deal with the mobilised toxins and rebuild your damaged tissues and immune system

• using fulvic acid and carbon-based binders to absorb and remove the toxins released when Lyme dies.

As well as:

- antimicrobial treatment (pharmaceutical or botanical) for Lyme
- an anti-inflammatory, nutrient-dense diet
- treatment of parasites (which can also harbour Lyme), co-infections, and other environmentally acquired illnesses such as heavy metal and mould toxicity that further compromise your immune system.

WHAT CAN I EXPECT WHEN I START TREATMENT?

Now that you have finally been diagnosed, you may feel relief at finally having a name for the multitude of symptoms you have been experiencing, but you may also be feeling daunted, and even angry that it took so long to diagnose and that few people took your suffering seriously along the way. This is completely normal.

No matter what treatment you decide to progress with, it is important to remember the following during your journey:

- There is not one set protocol for treating Lyme disease, and everyone's symptoms and response to treatment varies. Work with your practitioner to find what works for you.

- You will often feel worse before you feel better, because when Lyme bacteria dies, it releases endotoxins and inflammatory cytokines. The good news is that feeling worse means that treatment is working. However, if you are one of the lucky few that do not experience this, it doesn't mean your treatment isn't working! For more detailed information, see the details for Dr. Richard Horowitz's books at the end of this chapter.

Removing the dead borrelia bacteria and endotoxins as well as other toxins is critical. This can be done in many ways, such as through using binders, taking saunas or epsom salt and baking soda baths, and drinking lemon water.

HELPFUL REFERENCES AND RESOURCES

1. Horowitz, R.I.; Freeman, P.R. Efficacy of Double-Dose Dapsone Combination Therapy in the Treatment of Chronic Lyme Disease/Post-Treatment Lyme Disease Syndrome (PTLDS) and Associated Co-infections: A Report of Three Cases and Retrospective Chart Review. *Antibiotics* 2020, 9, 725. https://doi.org/10.3390/antibiotics9110725
Horowitz, R.I., Murali, K., Gaur, G. et al. Effect of dapsone alone and in combination with intracellular antibiotics against the biofilm form of B. burgdorferi. BMC Res Notes 13, 455 (2020).

2. Horowitz, Richard I M.D. 2017, *How Can I Get Better? An Action Plan for Treating Resistant Lyme and Chronic Disease*, St. Martin's Griffin, New York, New York, p 41-44

3. Dr. Horowitz's Sixteen-Point Differential Diagnosis MSIDS Map can be found in his book, Horowitz, Richard I M.D. 2017, *How Can I Get Better? An Action Plan for Treating Resistant Lyme and Chronic Disease*, St. Martin's Griffin, New York, New York, p 50-65

4. Validation of the Horowitz Multiple Systemic Infectious
   Disease Syndrome Questionnaire for Suspected Lyme Disease.
   Maryalice Citera*, Ph.D., Phyllis R. Freeman2, Ph.D., Richard
   I. Horowitz2, M.D., International Journal of General Medicine
   2017:10 249–273

https://www.dovepress.com/empirical-validation-of-the-horowitz-
multiple-systemic-infectious-dise-peer-reviewed-fulltext-article-
IJGM

http://www.ncbi.nlm.nih.gov/pubmed/28919803

The questionnaire can be found at: https://cangetbetter.com/
symptoms/

Dr. Richard Horowitz

Dr. Richard Horowitz, MD is one of the most sought out Lyme
Disease doctors in the world, and has 35 years' experience working
with patients with chronic infections. He is one of the founding
members of ILADS (the International Lyme & Associated Diseases
Society), the leader on Lyme Disease research and education.

Horowitz, Richard I M.D. 2013, *Why Can't I Get Better? Solving the
Mystery of Lyme and Chronic Disease*, St. Martin's Griffin, New York,
New York is his way of sharing his knowledge and experience in
treating chronic Lyme Disease.

Horowitz, Richard I M.D. 2017, *How Can I Get Better? An Action
Plan for Treating Resistant Lyme and Chronic Disease*, St. Martin's

Griffin, New York, New York is his latest Lyme book, and a national best seller.

His medical website provides more information on Lyme and tick-borne diseases: https://cangetbetter.com/symptoms/

His latest book, *Starseed R/evolution, The Awakening*, gives hope to those suffering with climate grief, as it provides novel solutions for our climate emergency.

www.microbeformulas.com

The Microbe Formulas website is my all-time favourite health resource for information on heavy metal toxicity, mould illness, parasites, Lyme disease and co-infections. On their site, Dr. Todd Watts and Dr. Jay Davidson of Microbe Formulas provide numerous videos and articles. You can search the Learn section by topic and find informative and enlightening resource materials as well as effective treatment and maintenance protocol advice. The support team at Microbe Formulas are fantastic. I called them many times to ask numerous questions about their products and treatment protocols, and I can't recommend them highly enough.

www.drjaydavidson.com

This website is also a treasure trove and has numerous articles about all aspects of Lyme disease. Dr. Jay Davidson, whose wife was seriously ill with Lyme for much of her life, is the co-founder of Microbe Formulas.

Dr. Jay's best-selling book, Davidson, J 2017, *How to Fix Lyme Disease: 3 Secrets to Improve Any Lyme Disease Treatment* CreateSpace Publishing, is a great resource. In this book, Dr. Jay gives you some of the best tips he has found to be game changers for those struggling with Lyme disease, in their path to healing.

www.buhnerhealing.com

Stephen Buhner was the first to do a comprehensive analysis of what Lyme disease does to the body and to develop herbal treatment protocols for Lyme and co-infections. He has written 23 books, including Buhner, S 2015 *'Healing Lyme: Natural Healing and Prevention of Lyme Borreliosis and Its Co-infections'*, Raven Press, which is considered by many to be an essential guide to Lyme and its treatment.

'THE MOST BEAUTIFUL PEOPLE ARE THOSE WHO HAVE KNOWN DEFEAT, KNOWN SUFFERING, KNOWN STRUGGLE, KNOWN LOSS, AND HAVE FOUND THEIR WAY OUT OF THE DEPTHS. THESE PERSONS HAVE AN APPRECIATION, A SENSITIVITY, AND AN UNDERSTANDING OF LIFE THAT FILLS THEM WITH COMPASSION, GENTLENESS, AND A DEEP LOVING CONCERN. BEAUTIFUL PEOPLE DO NOT JUST HAPPEN.'

ELIZABETH KUBLER ROS

CHAPTER EIGHT

TRAUMA
AN UNDERLYING FACTOR

FOR MANY YEARS, I KEPT HEARING THAT TRAUMA IS OFTEN AN UNDERLYING FACTOR IN CHRONIC ILLNESS, AND THAT WITH SERIOUS CONDITIONS LIKE LYME, HOLDING ONTO SUPPRESSED OR UNADDRESSED MAJOR TRAUMAS OR CLUSTERS OF MINOR TRAUMAS GETS IN THE WAY OF FULL HEALING.

I looked back at my happy childhood and thought, well, that doesn't apply to me. Then, I read a book about adoption called The Primal Wound, by Nancy Verrier, about how even when adoptees like me are raised in the most positive and loving environments, we are affected by the trauma that occurred when we were born. The penny finally dropped.

Nancy Verrier's research showed that bonding doesn't just begin after birth, it is a continuation of the physical, mental, and emotional bonding that begins in utero and continues throughout the post-natal period. Her book details how only being a few minutes or days old makes no difference to the level of trauma experienced when babies are removed from their biological mothers at birth and handed over to strangers. Not being able to remember it makes the trauma even more complicated, because although it cannot be recalled, the 'abandonment' and loss an adoptee experiences is indelibly imprinted on their limbic system and unconscious mind.

Her book resonated deeply with me. I finally understood that I had experienced a major trauma and was exhibiting the hallmarks of its impact on my physical health. Verrier explains how early trauma can impair regulation of your hypothalamic-pituitary-adrenocortical (HPA) axis. When someone's life begins with a trauma perceived to be 'life threatening', as it is for a baby taken from their mother, their cortisol and adrenaline levels rise dramatically, and their levels of serotonin drop. That becomes their normal biochemistry.

In this description of how this biochemical change becomes normal, I saw myself. I have a very high stress threshold, probably because I naturally produce high levels of stress hormones. My body effortlessly switches into 'high alert' mode during times of high stress, and although I feel and appear calm at the time, the high cortisol I produce wreaks havoc on my body, contributing to a cascade of symptoms at a later time. I have experienced this cycle of 'flares' many times over the past decade and finally realise that the adaptive strategy I developed the day I was born may not be serving my health well.

I certainly didn't blame anyone for my adoption and don't see myself as a victim. For me, love is what makes a family, and I had that in abundance. I had always known that my biological mother was only 16, and that she had given me up to give me a better life.

However, it was finally time to understand the impact, and that changing the physical patterns and sub-conscious belief systems that I had developed would help me to fully recover. Everyone has emotional wounds of some kind. When you hold onto suppressed and unaddressed trauma it affects your immune system, and your body will be less effective at fighting illness. If your body is stuck in 'fight or flight', it is harder for your body to digest, detoxify, and heal.

Therefore, it is essential to address any major trauma, or series of chronic traumas, that happened in your childhood so that you can fully heal and the wounds you experienced can stop being a stress on your body. There are many different effective trauma therapy techniques that can be used to heal from trauma, such as DNRS (Dynamic Neural Retraining System), EMDR (Eye Movement Desensitisation and Reprocessing), neurofeedback, somatic experiencing, EFT, and Cognitive Behavioural Therapy (CBT). As with any health issue, it is important to work with a qualified, experienced professional.

‘TRUE MENTAL
STRENGTH IS WHEN
YOU FIND FUEL IN AN
EMPTY TANK.’

UNKNOWN

CHAPTER NINE

CANCER
THE BIG ONE

JUST WHEN THE MICROBE FORMULAS TREATMENT PROTOCOL STARTED TO WORK, AND I WAS FEELING BETTER THAN I HAD IN YEARS, THERE WAS ONE MORE SURPRISE IN STORE.

Yep, the big C. The disease with the name that I wasn't even able to say out loud at first. The diagnosis that slapped me so hard that it sucked all the oxygen out of the air around me and brought me to my knees. In the days and weeks that followed, it snuck up on me when I least expected it and flooded my body with fear.

On New Year's Eve, 2020, I was diagnosed with Stage 3 breast cancer. I had an invasive, fast-growing, triple-negative tumour in my left breast that had spread to my axilla lymph nodes. It was going to require six months of chemotherapy and a mastectomy, followed by radiation therapy.

My heart broke like a glass hitting tiles, and the pieces were everywhere.

Over the next few weeks, as I was examined, scanned, biopsied, diagnosed, and given a treatment plan, I realised I needed better coping strategies. More than a decade of chronic illness had prepared me pretty well. I knew how to find strength when I was sure I didn't have any left, but this was a whole different situation. It felt on one hand like time was standing still, and on the other like I was being sucked into a giant swirling vortex. For the first time, I could understand why people don't go to the doctor when they know something is wrong, because once an illness is 'real', it can never be put it back in the box.

I read a quote from Desmond Tutu that resonated deeply: 'There is only one way to eat an elephant: one bite at a time.' To prevent being overwhelmed, I realised that I needed to break down what I was facing into pieces and only worry about one at a time. I also understood that I couldn't let my life stop for cancer. After diagnosis, when my manager suggested I take the next week off, I knew I needed to 'normalise' cancer into my life and not let it consume me. I needed the meaning and purpose that my work gave me. I had cancer, but it didn't have me.

One of the most difficult things I experienced during this time was sharing my diagnosis with loved ones. Their reactions reinforced the seriousness of what I was dealing with and scared me. Yet at the same time, feeling responsible for causing their pain, I found myself trying to offset their shock by reassuring them that I was okay and strong, instead of being honest about how frightened I really was.

When I talked to my doctor about this, she told me that the support I had during my treatment would be as important as the treatment itself, so I learned to reach out and be honest about what I was experiencing. Wrapping myself in the love and support that poured back was protective and comforting. Being able to trust my medical team helped enormously too. From the very beginning, their competence, their skill in compassionately delivering challenging news, and their acknowledgement of my concerns was reassuring.

When my doctor told me that cancer develops as a failure of your immune system, it all made sense. Usually, our immune system destroys cancer cells, but when it is overwhelmed, it cannot do so. The infections, pathogens, and toxins I had carried for so long had suppressed my immune system and helped create the conditions for my cancer to develop.

This set-back confirmed what I had learned years before: that healing is not linear. It is a 'two steps forward, one step back' journey, like doing the cha-cha. I realised that I still had a few rounds of the dance floor to do and strapped on my dance shoes. I had made enough progress that I was confident that my treatment protocol was working, and that I would eventually get better. But as well as treating the cancer itself, it was critical that I treat and remove the underlying cause(s) as well to reduce the chance of it ever coming back.

My cancer treatment tested me both mentally and physically in ways I could never have anticipated. The term 'post-traumatic growth' describes the positive personal changes that develop through a stressful or frightening experience. I developed new coping skills and more mental strength and felt empowered as a result. My connections with my family and friends deepened. Feelings of vulnerability led to my appreciating the beauty in the world around me even more. I added more spiritual depth to my life, and the things that really mattered became crystal clear. Hardship doesn't build character, it reveals it, and I will never again doubt how strong I am.

THE TIPS

'DON'T FORGET YOU'RE HUMAN. IT'S OKAY TO HAVE A MELTDOWN, JUST DON'T UNPACK AND LIVE THERE. CRY IT OUT AND THEN REFOCUS ON WHERE YOU ARE HEADED.'

UNKNOWN

CHAPTER TEN

TIPS FOR THE SUFFERER
HOW TO MAINTAIN YOUR SANITY WHEN YOU WANT TO JUST CURL UP AND GIVE UP

I OFTEN WONDER HOW I SURVIVED THE PAST 12 YEARS WITH MY SANITY INTACT AND HOW FOR MANY OF THOSE YEARS, I MANAGED TO EVEN KEEP MY JOB. IF I HAD KNOWN WHAT LAY AHEAD, I MIGHT HAVE GIVEN UP. THEY SAY THAT THE WORLD MUST BE ROUND SO THAT WE CAN'T SEE TOO FAR DOWN THE ROAD.

The biggest challenge for me was to maintain optimism and the belief that someday, I would suffer less. The fortitude and strength that I had to find to simply put one foot in front of the other on some days was enormous. My day often started with not knowing how I would get to its other end.

In addition, extreme gastrointestinal symptoms and sleep issues meant that I couldn't just curl up and binge on movies. My gut issues also meant that I couldn't eat any of the things that would normally bring comfort. The crushing exhaustion led to a hermit-like life, with little human interaction outside work and parenting.

Year after year, I set the goal of feeling better by the next Christmas, only to have to push that goal ahead again and again.

Over time, I found that one of the things that got me through was focussing on the things that made my life meaningful and brought me joy. On the days I suffered the most, doing something simple like making a nourishing dinner for my son gave me a sense of happiness and peace. In addition, a combination of naivety, grit, and determination to keep the train on the tracks got me through. But what made the whole experience easier was the compassion and support shown by my partner, David, whom I connected with in the last few years of being sick, when I was truly at my worst. His loving concern, patience in listening every day to my symptoms and struggles, and ability to always say something supportive and hopeful, got me through the darkest days.

In a world where many people would prefer not to have to go to work, my greatest wish was very simple. For me, being well meant I could actually go to work every day and contribute to the world around me in a significant and meaningful way. This was the light at the end of the tunnel for me.

I learned the following things over many years and after many failures, and they helped me to get through a journey that tested me in more ways than I ever thought possible.

MY TOP TIPS

Assemble an informed, compassionate team

During my health journey, I met some truly wonderful people in the medical community. Feeling as though they were working collaboratively with me helped enormously, because the partnerships you build with the people on your team is part of the medicine.

Taking an active role in your health will help you feel empowered. Seek out people who are happy to work collaboratively, such as doctors, integrative doctors, naturopaths, chiropractors, acupuncturists, and counsellors. You will need a whole team to get you through this. Ask around for recommendations. Use Facebook forums to get advice about who is good in your area, and don't be afraid to work with someone remotely.

Find reliable information about your illness(es), its treatment and management

This will help you feel you are taking a positive step and give you a feeling of control. But, be careful about your sources, sometimes too much information can be overwhelming and confusing.

Go low and slow with treatment

There is no magic pill for long-term illness. Recovery is a marathon, not a sprint. Long-term illnesses take a long time to resolve, and we can experience increased symptoms if we try to progress too quickly with treatment. As treatment progressed, I learned to see any new symptoms/diagnoses as a blessing, a red flag for something that still needed attention.

Develop skills and strategies to manage your symptoms

Finding ways to still my mind and calm my nervous system helped me handle the effects of my symptoms better. My strategies included the simplest of things such as taking a slow walk, a bath, noticing the beauty around me, and mindfulness.

Set small goals

It was important for me to have purpose even when I felt my worst. Setting goals, no matter how small, redirected my focus to the future and increased my resilience and hope. Sometimes my goals were as simple as increasing my medicine by a drop, or 1/8 tsp. over a week. Things as small as that helped me feel I was making progress.

Understand that recovery is not linear

I finally learned that an increase in symptoms was not necessarily a sign of failure to improve. It was important for me to understand that recovery often involves one step forward, then two steps back. I became able to accept setbacks without being afraid of them. I realised that speed doesn't matter, that forward is forward.

Write a symptom diary

People found it hard to understand that I didn't feel even a tiny bit better every day, like with the flu. At times, it has taken months before I could feel any noticeable progress. Being able to look back several months and see that there had been some progress was heartening. Keeping a symptom diary was helpful, as sometimes I would forget symptoms once they had disappeared. Seeing the overall list grow shorter gave me hope.

Find emotional support

You should never expect yourself to be able to handle the impact of a long-term illness on your own. Being so unwell often means that you rarely see friends or socialise in the ways you used to. It is so important that you speak to others who are going through what you are and to lean on family and friends when you need to. Asking for help is not a sign of weakness or failure. The support you have during your illness is an important part of what will help you get well.

In some cases, it may be good to find a counsellor to talk through certain aspects of your illness. Sometimes sharing the burden of the illness with friends or family is too heavy, and you find yourself reassuring them instead of being able to tell them how scared you are. There are things professionals will understand and be able to hear in a way your loved ones may not be able to.

Know that you don't always have to 'be positive'

There is often a lot of pressure when you are unwell to 'be positive', and the implication that if you aren't, your negativity will feed your illness. While it can help to be hopeful, this doesn't mean that you should deny the feelings that come with a serious or frightening illness. Trying to put on a brave face all the time will drain your energy and doesn't help you process any negative thoughts. Be realistic about what is happening, and talk to someone about your fears and concerns. Explaining how you feel to those around you may also help you receive the support you need.

Find gratitude

Some days it might be hard to find something to feel grateful for. That is understandable, but being grateful for even the simplest of things can help alleviate anxiety and help you see the light on the darkest days. If you only focus on the negative side of things, it can be hard to crawl out of that dark hole. Gratitude helps rewire and train your brain to see the positive side of things.

Acknowledge your grief

Everyone is human, and the emotions you feel are signposts for what you need. Long term illness comes with many losses. The way each person grieves is unique, but we all share the need for others to acknowledge our grief without trying to lessen or reframe it for us. If your grief is acknowledged, it will be much easier to move on from it.

If you can't see the light, be the light

When my symptoms are really bad, one of the things that always helps me feel better is by focussing on doing something for someone else. Making someone else's day brighter has the wonderful effect of making my own brighter at the same time.

Create a new reality

Belief and intention are incredibly powerful. Our perceptions can become a reality that we create for ourselves, so be aware of the reality you are creating. For instance, if you believe that you won't get better, you won't get better. It is so important that you set a positive intention, like 'I am going to heal, this is what I am going to do, and every day I will get better and better'. Don't worry about how. The intention itself is powerful enough to assist the process. If you continue to see yourself as a sick person, you will continue to be sick.

See the blessings that come from illness

When I finally found a doctor and team that I trusted and had a comprehensive diagnosis and clear treatment path, I began to trust that I was going to regain my health. Then I could see the gift I had been given through this experience — the opportunity to help others. Although I still had a few difficult years ahead, being able to see the blessings that had come from all this gave my life purpose and meaning.

Pace yourself

Pacing means managing your activity so that you don't wear yourself out. Limit your daily to-do list to only the essential tasks. Slow things down and take breaks. It may take longer, but you are more likely to finish the job without wearing yourself out. Schedule the most tiring tasks for when you have the most energy. Speak up and let people around you know when you need to stop. You are the one who will suffer if you are pushed beyond your limits. Set boundaries and say no. This sounds simple, but it can take practice - especially because on the days we feel good, we are so happy to not feel awful, we overdo it and then pay for it later.

Focus on today

The fear of the 'what ifs' used to almost paralyse me. What if I am getting sicker? What if I lose my job again? What if I can't pay my mortgage? Over time I learned that today was the only day I was dealing with. My philosophy became 'Get up, dress up, and show up'.

Focus on what you can control

Acknowledge that there are things that you can't control, but then move on and focus on what you can control, such as:

- where your focus is
- your reactions to situations
- where you spend and invest your time
- your self-talk and gratitude.

It is also important to:

- create a plan for managing your stress
- develop healthy affirmations/mantras that help you focus your thoughts in a positive way
- visualise and believe your goals
- identify the difference between ruminating and problem-solving, so you can avoid wasting time on unproductive thinking.

Keep asking questions

Trust your instincts. The more you feel you can trust the information and guidance you are being given, the more empowered you will feel. If your diagnosis does not fully explain your symptoms, if treatment isn't relieving them, keep asking questions. Remember that no question is silly. You deserve good answers and not to be made to feel you are questioning the intelligence of your treating doctor.

Understand that success is consistency

Integrating your treatment protocol into your daily routine and being consistent and persistent will ensure success.

Visualise the future – plant only what you want to harvest

Your thoughts can be very powerful. When you are chronically ill, often your attention is drawn to your symptoms. My day would often start with taking note of which symptoms were present and if there were any new ones, and scoring their severity.

I finally realised that focussing on them was reinforcing them and making me feel worse, that bemoaning my current situation was not helping me to create a different one. I started to nourish my mind with positive pictures. I visualised myself healthy and well, sitting on the beach, smiling. I focussed on how happy I felt, what the sun and wind felt like on my skin. This coping technique pulled me out of my pain, fear, and discomfort, and helped me feel relaxed and happy.

If you are having trouble finding what to focus on, here are a few suggestions you can try:

- a place that makes you feel relaxed and happy
- someone you love deeply
- something you like to do that makes you feel good.

If you find it difficult to focus, try a guided meditation.

Plan for the future

Recovering from complex, long-term illness is rarely a one-and-done experience. Maintaining good health often involves maintenance treatment and some long-term changes. Understand what you will need to do to maintain your health. You may need quarterly/annual periodic parasite, gut, or Lyme treatment to ensure you don't relapse. Genetic variations may mean that periodic detox is important. Discuss this with your practitioners, so you can be realistic about what you can expect with your future health and have a plan to manage it.

Join Facebook groups or other online forums

Be cautious. Anyone can say anything on the internet, but it doesn't make it true. But do look into the things that they suggest, because some of the people have done years of research and are very knowledgeable. Remember that the people who are posting are often those who have been sick for a long time and feel hopeless, so the majority of what you read might seem to be negative. There are many, many people who have successfully recovered who are busy living their active, healthy lives again.

Don't give up!

You will have difficult days, weeks, and maybe even months, especially the first few. Trust that every day, even though you may not feel it, you are moving a little bit closer to being well. You've got this.

'THE GREATEST GIFTS
ARE FOUND IN THE
HEARTS OF YOUR
LOVED ONES.'

UNKNOWN

CHAPTER ELEVEN

TIPS FOR YOUR LOVED ONES
TO HELP THOSE CLOSE TO YOU UNDERSTAND WHAT YOU NEED

YOU MIGHT FEEL ISOLATED DURING YOUR JOURNEY BACK TO HEALTH. DESPITE THEIR BEST EFFORTS, OUR LOVED ONES WILL FIND IT HARD TO UNDERSTAND THE CHALLENGES THAT COME WITH COMPLEX, LONG-TERM ILLNESS.

I know that watching me struggle for so long has been very difficult for my loved ones and the medical professionals who were trying to help. What the people around me said and how they reacted to my illness affected my journey both positively and negatively. The people close to you probably feel helpless and frustrated and might need guidance on what you need to hear and how they can support you through your journey.

At times I have found myself at a loss for the right thing to say to loved ones who were suffering, but I realise now that what they needed, like I did, was to hear simple, thoughtful, and supportive things like the ones below:

Hang in there

I found these three little words comforting. This simple expression of encouragement suggested to me that things would improve, and it helped me remain hopeful, persistent, and determined through challenging times.

You are not alone, I am here for you

I didn't enjoy being around myself when I felt really awful, so I couldn't imagine that anyone else wanted to be around me. I needed to hear that I was missed, and that people wanted to be around me. I needed them to make that extra effort to remind me that they were there for me when I was feeling up for it.

This sucks and is unfair

No one deserves chronic illness. I needed to be reminded that I deserved to be healthy and happy and that it must be rotten to experience this.

That must hurt/be uncomfortable/scary

There were so many symptoms I dealt with daily, but because my threshold was so high, I often didn't even mention them. When I did, it was because they were affecting me especially badly, and it helped when people didn't minimise or dismiss them and just acknowledged how crappy they must have been.

Tell me how you feel

It's difficult for anyone to know what to say in a situation they've never dealt with. Sometimes, it's not about what people say, but just that they sit and listen. All I needed was for people to say, "I don't know what to say, but I'm here for you".

You are so brave

I needed to be reminded of how strong I was and that it took strength and courage to keep fighting day after day.

You are doing an amazing job managing everything

A lot of the time it felt like it took ten times as much energy as usual to do normal things. Acknowledgement that I was managing to hold it all together despite feeling so unwell meant the world to me.

How can I help?

Most people find it difficult to ask for help. But that doesn't mean they don't want it and need it. This can be practical help or just lending an ear. Practical help can include:

- offering to do your shopping
- cooking a meal
- taking your kids somewhere for a few hours
- doing laundry
- cleaning the house
- taking you to appointments.

Tell me about your illness

I didn't like to bog people down by talking about my illness. The only way I felt comfortable talking about it was if people seemed interested. It helped when they asked me about my illness, how it felt, and how it affected my life.

You will get through this

Hearing this reassured me that although it felt like I was facing a mountain, eventually the load would lighten.

OTHER COMFORTING THINGS PEOPLE CAN SAY

- While I may not understand what you are going through, I am here if you need me.
- I'm sorry that you are going through this.
- I don't understand what you are going through, but I would like to know more.
- I wish I could take away your pain.
- I hope you feel better soon.
- It must be difficult to live with an illness which makes you feel so bad on the inside but doesn't show on the outside.

What not to say

- You complain a lot.
- Maybe you should get more exercise.
- You just need to be more positive.
- Do you think you are depressed?
- You don't look sick!
- Are you sure it's not all in your head?

Other tips

My loved ones found it easier to understand what I was experiencing if
I sent them well-written, credible articles or videos about my illnesses,
rather than if I just told them about it.

'JUST BECAUSE I
CARRY THE LOAD
WELL, DOESN'T MEAN
IT ISN'T HEAVY.'

UNKNOWN

TIPS FOR MEDICAL PROFESSIONALS AND HEALTH PRACTITIONERS TO HELP YOUR TREATING TEAM UNDERSTAND HOW TO BETTER SUPPORT YOU

MEDICAL PRACTITIONERS AND HEALTH PRACTITIONERS NEED TO UNDERSTAND THAT WE ARE MORE THAN THE ILLNESS WE WERE DIAGNOSED WITH, THAT WE ARE PEOPLE, WHO PROBABLY FEEL SCARED, OVERWHELMED, AND DISCOURAGED.

We want to feel cared about by the professionals who are treating us. When they show compassion, kindness, and support, we believe that our wellbeing is their priority, and that they have a genuine desire to help. This builds trust and can dramatically change our experience of our illness.

Here are some of the tips I have put together after 12 years of long-term illness. The medical and health professionals that I listed in my dedication do all these things, and their compassion and care helped make a very challenging experience so much better.

Compassion matters

Part of what was so distressing about my journey to regain my health was the stress and trauma of dealing with medical professionals who were dismissive and closed-minded. There is so much more to being a good medical professional than accurately interpreting diagnostic tests, maintaining technical competency, and prescribing treatment. I wish had a dollar for every time a medical professional looked at me after I explained my medical history and symptoms and said, with a sceptical tone, 'But you look healthy'.

Don't rush me out the door

Feeling like you have taken the time to hear me is comforting. I understand there are limits to how much of your time I can have, but if we haven't had enough time, please suggest I book a longer/ double appointment next time.

Acknowledge my suffering

A simple and effective thing to say is 'Good to see you. I'm sorry, it sounds like you've had a tough, tough week.' Be aware that your tone of voice can have a huge impact.

Listen

It helps if I feel like you take me and my symptoms seriously. Take the time to ask me questions about what I am experiencing and whether I have any questions.

Be open-minded

I read somewhere that 90% of patients with a long-term illness will know more about it than their treating doctors. That is because we research exhaustively, trying to find anything that might give us answers. We belong to forums where we talk with people all over the world, and gain knowledge. If I bring research to you, and it includes information you have not come across before, please show interest and don't automatically dismiss it because you have not heard of it. It may be emerging thinking that is quite useful, and will become mainstream someday.

Don't be afraid to admit you don't have all the answers

I respected the doctors who admitted that they didn't have the answers to some of my questions, but showed interest in helping me find them. Honesty built trust, and trust is key in a good patient/doctor relationship.

Help me understand what to expect along the way

Having an idea of what symptoms I might expect, and how I could offset them, helped me mentally and practically prepare for them.

Help cultivate and maintain hope

Hearing things like, 'I will do everything I can to help you', from medical professionals was enormously reassuring, and helped to reduce my feelings of stress.

'SOMETIMES THE THINGS WE CAN'T CHANGE END UP CHANGING US.'

UNKNOWN

CONCLUSION

THIS IS THE BOOK I WISH I HAD READ 12 YEARS AGO, AND THE ONE I PROMISED MYSELF I WOULD WRITE WHEN I HAD RECOVERED FROM OVER A DECADE OF MYSTERIOUS AND DEBILITATING SYMPTOMS THAT NO ONE COULD EXPLAIN, AND WHEN I WAS FINALLY A SUCCESS STORY. I HOPE THAT IT HAS HELPED YOU GAIN THE KNOWLEDGE OF HOW YOU CAN ALSO GET WELL, AND THAT IT HELPS YOU BELIEVE THAT YOU CAN.

For years, I dreamed of being like Brenda Cosentino, whose blog I had discovered. She had recovered her health after suffering from Lyme disease, chronic fatigue, and fibromyalgia for over 20 years and was climbing ruins in Mexico. I so desperately wanted that to be me. I had been struggling for so long that being active and healthy was a distant memory, but I could still recall how it felt and was determined to find answers that would allow me to feel that way again.

Over a period of twelve years, I saw over forty different doctors, medical professionals, and specialists and spent over $150,000 on appointments and supplements. My life consisted of managing the symptoms that dominated every day. It was overwhelming, difficult, and harrowing at times. I was exhausted from trying to keep the train on the tracks.

Looking back, I find it hard to fathom how I made it through. By the time I was properly diagnosed, my world was very small.

My life felt so different from those around me because there were so many things I wasn't able to do. My doctor calls Lyme disease 'the marriage buster', and I can see why. It took all my energy to be a mom and to work, so there wasn't much left for nurturing friendships or intimate relationships.

My determination and search for answers paid off. After being diagnosed with Lyme disease, I listened to the entire online Chronic Lyme Disease Summit in July 2020 and became aware of Dr. Richard Horowitz, Dr. Jay Davidson, and Dr. Todd Watts and their work. I finally found the answer to my chronic health issues. From these doctors, I learned that chronic illness is never about just one specific infection or illness. Regaining my health didn't happen overnight, but it did happen. This can also happen for you. Believe that you can also recover when you clear the toxins, pathogens, and infections that are affecting your immune system.

Adversity never leaves us as it found us, and now that I have recovered, I can see the positive ways that the journey has changed me. In particular, I have become more compassionate. I can more easily sense when other people around me are struggling, and I now understand how to support them better. As they say, you don't bounce back from difficult times, you bounce forward.

There is hope. Hang in there and keep going, surround yourself with a good support team, and never give up. You will get there - I am proof of that.

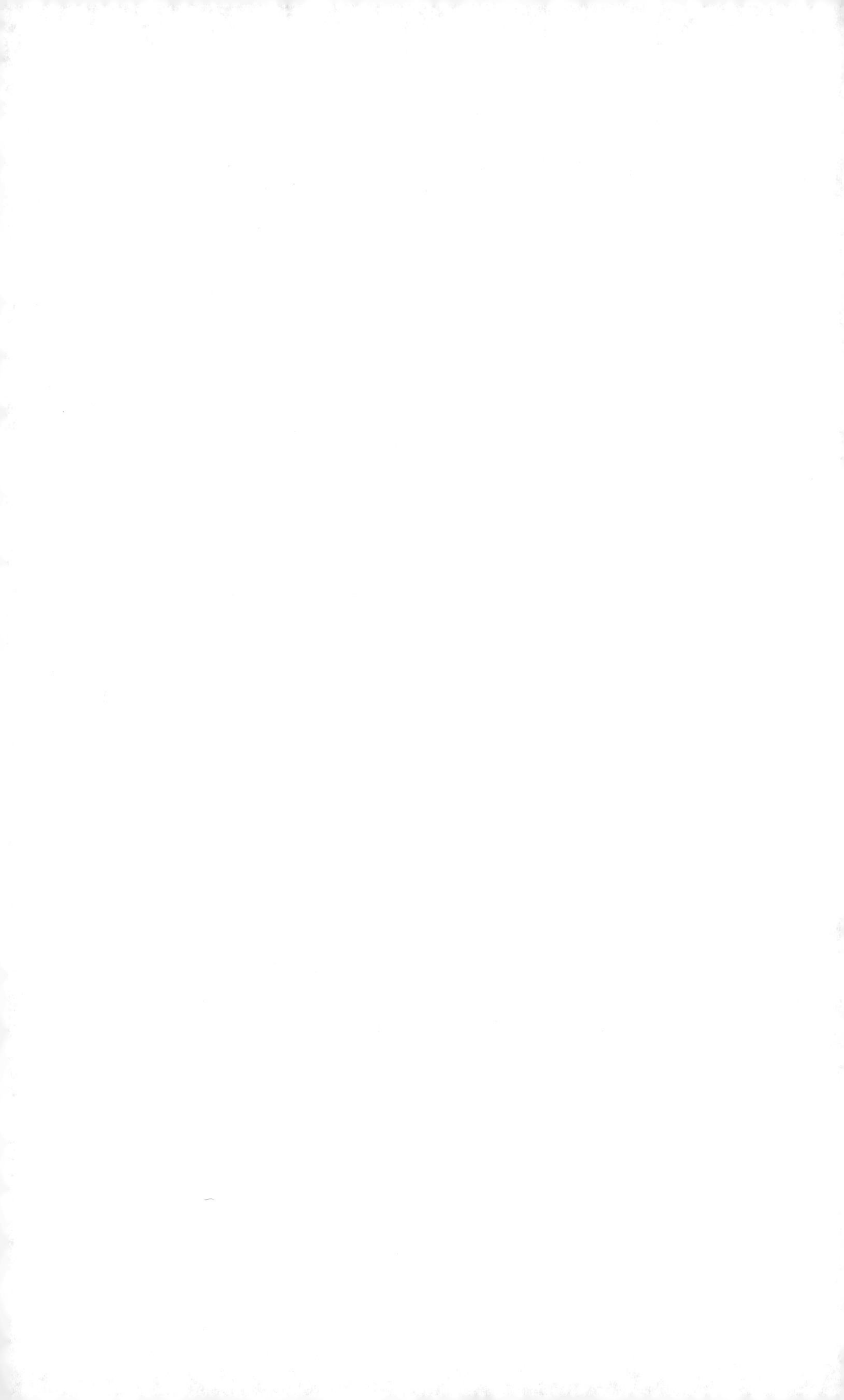